KSL
M000302085

PTCE AND EXCPT PREP

400 MEDICATIONS
SIMPLIFIED

MEMORIZE FASTER
PASS WITH CONFIDENCE

RYAN NGOV, PHARMD

Reshape The Mind, Inc.
1319 Alpine Cir.
Baldwin Park, CA 91706
www.reshapethemind.com

Copyright © 2020 by Ryan Ngov

All rights reserved. No part of this book may be reproduced, stored in retrieval system, or transmitted in any form or by any means electronic, mechanical, photocopying, recording, or otherwise without prior written permission of the publisher and the author. For information, contact Reshape The Mind, Inc. at support@reshapethemind.com

The information contained in this book is for general education purposes only. While the information contained in this book is intended to be accurate at the time of publishing, nothing should be construed as legal, tax, financial, or medical advice.

Printed in the United States of America

Library of Congress Control Number: 2020918540

ISBN 978-1-970084-04-7 (Paperback)
ISBN 978-1-970084-05-4 (Mobi)
ISBN 978-1-970084-06-1 (Epub)

First Edition October 2020

10 9 8 7 6 5 4 3

CONTENTS

INTRODUCTION

4*00 Medications Simplified* is designed to help students quickly memorize the most commonly prescribed medications in the United States, specifically their generic and brand names, pharmacologic classes, and indications. That's it. The book is therefore a supplement (not a replacement) to augment either a formalized pharmacy technician training program or on-the-job training.

Whether you are a nursing student, premed, pre-pharm, or an aspiring pharmacy technician preparing for the PTCE or the ExCPT exam, this book will introduce you to how seemingly nonsensical medication names can be organized meaningfully so that one can recall them at will. Again, this book is not comprehensive by nature as it merely addresses the aforementioned four components.

Besides the featured top 300 medications, an additional 100 is preserved in Part 4 for those who are keen to learn more, those who are motivated to outwork others, and those who want to differentiate themselves from the crowd in the competitive job market.

The strength of this book lies in the medication organization, which facilitates the memorization process. The alphabetical order of both generic and brand names promotes quick access to any medication. Details such as drug dosing, mechanism of action, adverse drug event, contraindications, etc. are not discussed here to prevent information overload. All those details can be found in other reference materials mentioned in the References section.

Content Coverage for PTCE and ExCPT Exam

———— ❧ ————

The tables below outline the knowledge domain of PTCE and ExCPT exam. It also indicates the content that this book will cover with regards to those requirements.

Overview of PTCE Requirements and what this book covers

Knowledge domains	Domain description	% PTCE Content
1*	Medications	40
2	Federal regulations	12.5
3	Patient safety and quality assurance	26.25
4	Order entry and processing	21.25

*This book only covers parts of the Medications domain, as elaborated in the next table.

Detailed Medications subdomains of PTCE and what this book covers

Knowledge Domains and Areas		% of PTCE Exam Content
1.	**Medications**	**40%**
1.1**	Generic names, brand names, and classifications of medications	
1.2	Therapeutic equivalence	
1.3	Common and life-threatening drug interactions and contraindications	
1.4	Strengths/dose, dosage forms, routes of administration, special handling and administration instructions, and duration of drug therapy	
1.5	Common and severe medication side effects, adverse effects, and allergies	
1.6**	Indications of medications and dietary supplements	
1.7	Drug stability	
1.8	Narrow therapeutic index (NTI) medications	
1.9	Physical and chemical incompatibilities related to non-sterile compounding and reconstitution	
1.10	Proper storage of medications	

**This book covers part 1.1 and 1.6 under the Medications domain.

Summary ExCPT Exam Outline and what this book covers

Domain	# of Items on Exam
1. Overview and Laws	**25**
A. Role, scope of practice, and general duties of the pharmacy technician	11
B. Laws and regulations	8
C. Controlled substances	6
2. Drugs and drug therapy***	**15**
A. Drug classification	9
B. Frequently prescribed medications	6
3. Dispensing Process	**45**
A. Prescription and medication order	15
B. Intake and entry preparing and dispensing prescriptions	13
C. Calculations	7
D. Sterile and nonsterile products, compounding, unit dose, and repackaging	10
4. Medication safety and quality assurance	**15**
Total	100

*** This book covers Drug and drug therapy section of the ExCPT. Again, this book only addresses four components of drug: generic name, brand name, pharmacologic class, and indication.

FREQUENTLY ASKED QUESTIONS

How is this book different from others in the market?

With its minimalist approach, this book eliminates unnecessary information about these medications to enable students to laser focus on the critical task at hand, which is to memorize all the medications as quickly as possible. It is also organized in ways that have been scientifically proven to enhance medication memorization. The extra 100 medications are preserved in Part 4 for the students motivated to learn more.

Why 400 medications?

This book is written for those who want to master the top 300 medications quickly and those who want the option to go above and beyond. The extra 100 medications are presented in a different section of the book so they will not interfere with those who do not have the time or intention to learn more than necessary. As the pharmacy field is becoming increasingly competitive, some students see the benefits of overpreparation for their future careers. Should you wish to outwork your competition, this book has you covered. Besides, increasing your competence is a great way to increase your confidence.

Why do I need this book?

This book was written for students who do not have much time to prepare for the PTCE or the ExCPT exam but wish to optimize their medication memorization process with minimal effort.

Why should people pay for this book when they can get similar stuff for FREE from the internet?

FREE stuff on the internet is usually unreliable for many reasons. First and foremost, there is no proper or respectable source of reference for the information provided. Secondly, the author tends to be unverifiable and therefore not trustworthy with the materials they share. Furthermore, the medications are not well organized to help students with their memorization process. Students actually PAY a price indirectly by putting effort and time into organizing the material themselves. By contrast, this book was created with the intention of helping students to learn quickly and thereby optimize the use of their time.

Where do those extra one hundred medications come from?

The top 300 medications from the previous three consecutive years were collected and compared to the most recent top-prescribed medications in the United States. The medications that were no longer ranked in the top 300 were reviewed and picked based on their past ranking and the author's personal experience working in the retail pharmacy setting.

If I just want to get a pharmacy technician license, do I have to take the PTCE or the ExCPT exam?

No, you don't have to. Details on how to get a license without taking the PTCE or the ExCPT are provided in the section "WAYS TO GET A PHARMACY TECH LICENSE".

What are some of the advantages of having a CPhT credential?

With that credential, you could apply for a pharmacy technician license in many states and therefore increase your mobility. Other benefits include: more job opportunities, better salary, professional designation (CPhT), proven clinical knowledge, demonstrated commitment to the field, and increased opportunities for advancement.

What is the difference between a CPhT credential and a pharmacy technician license?

The main difference is that a license is a required component to work as a pharmacy technician, whereas a CPhT credential is not. A pharmacy technician license can be obtained with or without a CPhT credential. A CPhT credential allows you to apply for the license in many states.

HOW TO USE THIS BOOK

To get started, go over the Memorization Tips given in the next section. Part 1 is probably the most important section as it groups the medications under the same pharmacologic class for the treatment of a particular disease state. This should facilitate learning as it gives meaning to those otherwise meaningless generic/brand medications.

While Part 2 has all the top 300 generic medications sorted in alphabetical order, Part 3 has all the brand medications arranged in the same fashion. For students who only aim to pass their PTCE or ExCPT, you may skip Part 4, which contains 100 bonus medications preserved for those with extra time or motivation to learn more and get ahead of others.

Part 5 of the book is where you can practice what you have learned. Although the tables merely have a blank column for you to write the generic or brand name of a medication, you may further test yourself with regards to their pharmacologic classes and even their indications.

MEMORIZATION TIPS

———— ⚜ ————

We all have our own stories and struggles when it comes to memorization. Many people were even convinced that they had a bad memory at some point in their lives! Fortunately, that was a lie. Unless you were born with a certain genetic or mental defect, there is no such thing as a good or bad memory, only a trained or untrained memory. In other words, our memory is a trainable skillset that can get better over time if we constantly work on it. I am by no means a memory expert, but I have put together a few time-tested memorization techniques from the books I have read, memory experts on the subject matter like Kevin Horsley, and my own experience going through a pharmacy school.

Learning is the process of connecting what we already know to something new. The definition of a vocabulary or the translation of a foreign term are examples of how we learn (by connecting the known to the unknown). We learn the name of a medication (unknown at first) by remembering what it is used for (the known disease state or indication). This learning fundamental is the key to mastering the power of our incredible and creative mind to remember.

4 Steps to Memory Expansion

These four steps mastering series involves Kevin Horsley's "**SEE**" Principle that stands for **S**enses, **E**xaggeration, and **E**nergize. The fourth step is the **S**torage compartment. We will use **SEES** to represent the series.

- **STEP 1 (Senses):** There are five senses (sight, sound, smell, touch, and taste) that we use daily to perceive any information. The more senses we can attach to a particular object or medication, the more vivid our memory of that object/medication will be.

- **STEP 2 (Exaggeration):** When we make something larger, better, or worse than it really is, we create more vivid images in our brain and that serves to make the memory last longer! For example, a normal-size orange is less memorable than one that is as huge as a house.

- **STEP 3 (Energize):** By making a still object move, we give it energy and life! If an orange could talk, run, or dance, that would make it easier to remember as compared to a still orange.

- **STEP 4 (Storage):** Once you have applied the SEE Principle, you need a familiar storage compartment in which to keep those mental images or movies. The storage compartment enables quick access to stored items in any order. Some common storage that people can easily navigate in their minds are their cars, the human body parts, and different rooms (bedroom, bathroom, kitchen, living room, etc.) in a house.

It has been found that the more ridiculous the mental images or mind-movies we create, the longer they will last in our memory. As the four steps mastering series is not intuitive or normally practiced, it will require some effort at the beginning. Once you get familiar with the techniques, you will notice the rapid expansion of your memory capacity. It is important to remember that practice makes progress and that if we don't use it, we will lose it.

Additional Study Guide

B elow are extra memorization tips to help you master all the medications you need to know for the PTCE or ExCPT exam:

1. **ENVIRONMENT**: Select an environment that is conducive to your learning style. While many people thrive in places with minimal distractions, like a quiet room, some students find better luck in public areas, such as a library or coffee shop.

2. **MEDICATION CLASS:** Medications within the same class share similar functions and generic names. For example, beta blockers are used for hypertension and they share the stem "-olol" (Metoprolol, Atenolol, Propranolol) while proton pump inhibitors are used for acid reflux and share the stem "-prazole" (Omeprazole, Pantoprazole).

3. **SMALL GROUP:** Instead of going over 300+ medications in one setting, try breaking them into smaller groups of 20 to 30 medications. This makes it less overwhelming and more manageable.

4. **DAILY SCHEDULE:** Schedule a certain amount of time per day to sit down and go over each group of the medications you plan to memorize. A 30-minute session is usually sufficient. Master two or more groups of medications if you feel highly motivated or if your test is around the corner.

5. **PRACTICE ROUTINE:** Establish a routine to review older material. For example, before hitting on a new group of medications you plan to memorize, make sure to first go over the ones you have learned the previous day or session.

6. **SPACED REPETITION**: Apply the spaced repetition principle to help commit those medications to your long-term memory. Spaced repetition refers to revisiting or rereading the same medications at a planned interval, such as one or two hours after your first attempt to memorize them. The use

of an alarm clock to set reminders has been proven to be particularly useful for this strategy.

7. **BE PROACTIVE**: Get proactive by making flashcards in your own handwriting. You may fill a flashcard with one medication or all the medications under the same class or disease state, including its respective brand name(s) and indication on the opposite side. The use of different color pens/markers for different classes of medications is super effective as it makes a longer-lasting impression.

8. **SLEEP**: Getting enough sleep at night tremendously improves your memory and concentration level. At least seven hours of sleep per day is recommended for most people.

9. **RINSE AND REPEAT**: Repeat step one through eight until you have completely memorized all the medications.

PART 1

TYPES OF DISORDERS

1.

BONE AND JOINT

This chapter covers the following disease states:

1. Rheumatoid Arthritis

2. Osteoporosis

3. Gout.

The pharmacologic classes used are:

1. Disease-modifying antirheumatic drugs (DMARDs)

2. Bisphosphonate

3. Uricosuric Agent

4. Xanthine Oxidase Inhibitor.

Rheumatoid Arthritis

CLASS: Disease-modifying antirheumatic drugs (DMARDs)		
GENERIC	**BRAND**	**OTHER INDICATION**
Adalimumab	Humira	Psoriatic Arthritis, Crohn Disease, Ulcerative Colitis
Methotrexate	Trexall	Psoriasis, Cancer, Neoplasms, Leukemia
Cyclosporine	Neoral, Sandimmune, Gengraf	Psoriasis, Solid Organ Transplantation
Hydroxychloroquine	Plaquenil	Lupus, Malaria

Osteoporosis

CLASS: Bisphosphonate	
GENERIC	**BRAND**
Alendronate	Fosamax

Gout

GENERIC	**BRAND**	**CLASS**
Colchicine	Colcrys	**Uricosuric Agent**
Allopurinol	Zyloprim	**Xanthine Oxidase Inhibitor**

2.

CARDIOVASCULAR

The disease states covered by this chapter are:

1. Hypertension

2. Arrhythmias

3. Stroke

4. Deep Vein Thrombosis

5. Angina

6. Acute Coronary Syndromes

7. Cholesterol

8. Edema

9. Heart Attack

10. Septic Shock

11. Anaphylaxis

The pharmacologic classes that are used include

1. Angiotensin-converting enzyme inhibitor

2. Angiotensin II Receptor Blocker

3. Beta Blocker

4. Calcium Channel Blocker (CCB)

5. α2-Adrenergic Agonist

6. Peripheral Vasodilator

7. Antiarrhythmic

8. Anticoagulant

9. Antihyperlipidemic

10. Diuretic

11. Antianginal, and

12. Anaphylaxis Agent.

Hypertension

| CLASS: Angiotensin-converting enzyme (ACE) Inhibitor ||
GENERIC	BRAND
Benazepril	Lotensin
Benazepril + Amlodipine	Lotrel
Enalapril	Vasotec
Lisinopril	Prinivil, Zestril
Lisinopril + HCTZ	Zestoretic
Quinapril	Accupril
Ramipril	Altace

| CLASS: Angiotensin II Receptor Blocker (ARB) ||
GENERIC	BRAND
Irbesartan	Avapro
Losartan	Cozaar
Losartan + HCTZ	Hyzaar
Olmesartan	Benicar
Olmesartan + HCTZ	Benicar HCT
Telmisartan	Micardis
Valsartan	Diovan
Valsartan + HCTZ	Diovan HCT

| CLASS: Beta Blocker ||
GENERIC	BRAND
Atenolol	Tenormin
Atenolol + Chlorthalidone	Tenoretic
Bisoprolol	Zebeta
Carvedilol	Coreg
Labetalol	Normodyne
Metoprolol	Toprol XL, Lopressor
Nebivolol	Bystolic
Propranolol	Inderal

| CLASS: Calcium Channel Blocker (CCB) ||
GENERIC	BRAND
Amlodipine	Norvasc
Diltiazem	Cardizem, Cartia XT
Nifedipine	Procardia, Adalat
Verapamil	Calan SR

| CLASS: α2-Adrenergic Agonist ||
GENERIC	BRAND
Clonidine	Catapres
Guanfacine	Intuniv

| CLASS: Peripheral Vasodilator ||
GENERIC	BRAND
Hydralazine	Apresoline

Arrhythmias

| CLASS: Antiarrhythmic ||
GENERIC	BRAND
Amiodarone	Cordarone
Digoxin	Lanoxin
Flecainide	Tambacor
Sotalol	Betapace, Sorine

Stroke, Deep Vein Thrombosis, Angina, Acute Coronary Syndromes

| CLASS: Anticoagulant ||
GENERIC	BRAND
Apixaban	Eliquis
Rivaroxaban	Xarelto
Enoxaparin	Lovenox
Warfarin	Coumadin
Clopidogrel	Plavix

Cholesterol

| CLASS: Antihyperlipidemic ||
GENERIC	BRAND
Ezetimibe	Zetia
Ezetimibe + Simvastatin	Vytorin
Niacin	Niaspan, Slo-Niacin
Omega-3 Fatty Acid Ethyl Esters	Lovaza
Fenofibrate	Tricor, Trilipix
Gemfibrozil	Lopid
Atorvastatin	Lipitor
Lovastatin	Mevacor
Pravastatin	Pravachol
Rosuvastatin	Crestor
Simvastatin	Zocor

Edema

| CLASS: Diuretic ||
GENERIC	BRAND
Bumetanide	Bumex, Burinex
Furosemide	Lasix
Torsemide	Demadex
Spironolactone	Aldactone
Hydrochlorothiazide (HCTZ)	Microzide
Hydrochlorothiazide (HCTZ) + Triamterene	Dyazide, Maxzide
Chlorthalidone	Hygroton, Thalitone

*Hydrochlorothiazide, Hydrochlorothiazide + Triamterene, and Chlorthalidone are mainly used for hypertension. They are put here in the diuretic class table under edema for the purpose of easy memorization.

Angina

CLASS: Antianginal	
GENERIC	BRAND
Ranolazine	Ranexa
Isosorbide Mononitrate	Imdur
Nitroglycerin	Nitrostat, Minitran

Heart Attack, Hypotension Associated with Septic Shock, Anaphylaxis

CLASS: Anaphylaxis Agent	
GENERIC	BRAND
Epinephrine Auto-Injector	Drenaclick, Auvi-Q, EpiPen, EpiPen Jr

3.

DERMATOLOGIC

The disease states covered in this chapter are: Acne Vulgaris, Inflammation, Psoriasis, and Skin Infection. The following pharmacologic classes used are: Topical Retinoids, Antibiotic, Antifungal, and Corticosteroid.

Acne Vulgaris

CLASS: Topical Retinoids	
GENERIC	BRAND
Tretinoin	Retin A

Antibiotic	
GENERIC	BRAND
Ciprofloxacin	Cipro
Erythromycin	Erythrocin
Doxycycline	Vibramycin
Minocycline	Dynacin, Minocin, Solodyn
Sulfamethoxazole + Trimethoprim	Bactrim

Inflammation, Psoriasis

CLASS: Corticosteroid		
GENERIC	BRAND	INDICATION
Clobetasol	Impoyz, Temovate	Psoriasis
Hydrocortisone Topical	Cortisone	Inflammation
Triamcinolone Topical	Kenalog, Trianex, Triacet	Inflammation
Betamethasone Dipropionate + Clotrimazole	Lotrisone	Tinea Cruris, Tinea Corporis, Tinea Pedis

Topical Products for Infection

GENERIC	BRAND	CLASS
Bacitracin + Neomycin + Polymyxin B	Neosporin	Antibiotic
Mupirocin	Bactroban	Antibiotic
Nystatin	Mycostatin, Nyamyc, Nystop	Antifungal
Ketoconazole Topical	Nizoral	Antifungal

4.

ENDOCRINOLOGIC

This chapter covers these disease states: Diabetes, Hypothyroidism, and Hyperthyroidism. The pharmacologic classes used are: Antidiabetic, Thyroid, and Thioureas.

Diabetes

CLASS: Antidiabetic		
GENERIC	**BRAND**	**SUBCLASS**
Metformin	Glucophage	Biguanides
Metformin + Sitagliptin	Janumet XR	Biguanides + Dipeptidyl Peptidase-4 Inhibitor
Sitagliptin	Januvia	Dipeptidyl Peptidase 4 Inhibitor
Linagliptin	Tradjenta	Dipeptidyl Peptidase 4 Inhibitor
Insulin Degludec	Tresiba	Insulin, Long Acting
Insulin Detemir	Levemir	Insulin, Long Acting
Insulin Glargine	Lantus	Insulin, Long Acting
Insulin Aspart	Novolog	Insulin, Rapid Acting
Insulin Lispro	Humalog, Novolog	Insulin, Rapid Acting
Insulin Human	Humulin R, Novolin R	Insulin, Short Acting
Empagliflozin	Jardiance	Sodium-glucose cotransporter 2 inhibitor
Canagliflozin	Invokana	Sodium-glucose cotransporter 2 inhibitor

Dapagliflozin	Farxiga	Sodium-glucose cotransporter 2 inhibitor
Glimepiride	Amaryl	Sulfonylureas
Glipizide	Glucotrol	Sulfonylureas
Glyburide	Micronase, Diabeta	Sulfonylureas
Pioglitazone	Actos	Thiazolidinediones
Dulaglutide	Trulicity	Glucagon-Like Peptide-1 Receptor Agonist
Exenatide	Byetta, Bydureon	Glucagon-Like Peptide-1 Receptor Agonist
Liraglutide	Victoza, Saxenda	Glucagon-Like Peptide-1 Receptor Agonist

Hypothyroidism

CLASS: Thyroid	
GENERIC	**BRAND**
Levothyroxine	Synthroid
Liothyronine	Cytomel
Thyroid	Armour Thyroid

Hyperthyroidism

CLASS: Thioureas	
GENERIC	**BRAND**
Methimazole	Tapazole

5.

GASTROINTESTINAL

The disease states covered under gastrointestinal disorder are

1. Motion Sickness

2. Nausea and Vomiting

3. Constipation

4. Cough

5. Gastroesophageal Reflux Disease (GERD)

6. Ulcerative Colitis

7. Pancreatic Insufficiency, and

8. Irritable Bowel Sndrome (IBS).

The pharmacologic classes used are:

1. Antiemetic, Laxative

2. Antitussive

3. Proton Pump Inhibitor

4. Histamine H2 Antagonist

5. Mucosal Protectant

6. 5-Aminosalicylic Acid Derivatives

7. Pancreatic/Digestive Enzyme, and

8. Anticholinergic.

Motion Sickness, Nausea and Vomiting

| CLASS: Antiemetic ||
GENERIC	BRAND
Mesalamine	Asacol
Ondansetron	Zofran
Metoclopramide	Reglan
Promethazine	Phenergan
Meclizine	Antivert, Bonine, Dramamine

Constipation

| CLASS: Laxative ||
GENERIC	BRAND
Docusate Sodium	Colace
Methylcellulose	Citrucel
Polyethylene Glycol 3350	Miralax
Sennosides	Senna, Senokot
Linaclotide	Linzess

Cough

| CLASS: Antitussive ||
GENERIC	BRAND
Benzonatate	Tessalon Perles
Guaifenesin	Mucinex
Guaifenesin + Pseudoephedrine + Codeine	Cheratussin DAC, Virtussin DAC

Gastroesophageal Reflux Disease (GERD)

CLASS: Proton Pump Inhibitor	
GENERIC	**BRAND**
Dexlansoprazole	Dexilant
Esomeprazole	Nexium
Lansoprazole	Prevacid
Omeprazole	Prilosec
Rabeprazole	Aciphex
Pantoprazole	Protonix

CLASS: Histamine H2 Antagonist	
GENERIC	**BRAND**
Famotidine	Pepcid
Ranitidine	Zantac

CLASS: Mucosal Protectant	
GENERIC	**BRAND**
Sucralfate	Carafate

Other Classes Under Gastrointestinal Disorders

GENERIC	BRAND	CLASSIFICATION	INDICATION
Mesalamine	Asacol	5-Aminosalicylic Acid Derivatives	Ulcerative Colitis
Pancrelipase	Creon, Zenpep	Pancreatic/Digestive Enzyme	Pancreatic Insufficiency
Dicyclomine	Bentyl	Anticholinergic	Irritable Bowel Sndrome (IBS) / Abdominal Cramps

6.

GYNECOLOGIC

This chapter covers Birth Control, Menopause, and Abnormal Uterine Bleeding. The pharmacologic classes used are Contraceptive, Menopausal Hormone Therapy, and Progestogen.

Birth Control

CLASS: Contraceptive	
GENERIC	BRAND
Ethinyl Estradiol + Desogestrel	Apri, Cyclessa, Enskyce, Viorele
Ethinyl estradiol + Drospirenone	Yaz
Ethinyl Estradiol + Etonogestrel	NuvaRing
Ethinyl Estradiol + Levonorgestrel	Twirla
Ethinyl Estradiol + Norethindrone	Necon 777
Ethinyl Estradiol + Norgestimate	Trinessa-28, Ortho Tri-Cyclen, Ortho Tri-Cyclen Lo
Ethinyl Estradiol + Norgestrel	Cryselle
Norethindrone	Errin, Heather, Camila

Menopause

| CLASS: Menopausal Hormone Therapy ||
GENERIC	BRAND
Estradiol oral	Estrace
Estrogens, Conjugated	Premarin
Conjugated Estrogens + Medroxyprogesterone	Prempro

Abnormal Uterine Bleeding

| CLASS: Progestogen ||
GENERIC	BRAND
Progesterone	Prometrium
Medroxyprogesterone	Provera, Depo-Provera

7.

⸺⸻᯼⸻⸺

HEMATOLOGIC

This chapter only cover Anemias and the pharmacologic class used is Vitamins.

Anemias

CLASS: Vitamins	
GENERIC	**BRAND**
Ferrous Sulfate	Feosol, Fer-In-Sol
Cyanocobalamin	Vitamin B12
Folic Acid	Folate, Folvite

8.

❦

INFECTIOUS DISEASES

This chapter covers Infection and Transplant. The pharmacologic classes used are: Antibiotic, Antifungal, Antiviral, and Immunosuppressant.

Infection

CLASS: Antibiotic	
GENERIC	**BRAND**
Amoxicillin	Amoxil
Amoxicillin + Clavulanate	Augmentin
Cefdinir	Omnicef
Cephalexin	Keflex
Clindamycin	Cleocin
Nitrofurantoin	Macrobid, Macrodantin
Levofloxacin	Levaquin
Azithromycin	Z-Pak, Zithromax
Penicillin VK	Pen Vee K, Penicillin V
Chlorhexidine	Peridex, PerioGard, PerioChip

CLASS: Antifungal	
GENERIC	**BRAND**
Fluconazole	Diflucan
Metronidazole	Flagyl

CLASS: Antiviral	
GENERIC	**BRAND**
Acyclovir	Zovirax
Valacyclovir	Valtrex
Oseltamivir	Tamiflu
Emtricitabine	Emtriva

Transplant (Heart, Liver, Kidney)

CLASS: Immunosuppressant	
GENERIC	**BRAND**
Mycophenolate	CellCept, Myfortic

9.

⚬❦⚬

NEUROLOGIC

This chapter covers the following disease states:

1. Alzheimer

2. Parkinson

3. Seizure

4. Anxiety

5. Muscle Spasm

6. Pain Management

7. Migraine Headache.

The pharmacologic classes used are:

1. Central Cholinesterase Inhibitor

2. N-methyl-D-aspartate (NMDA) Receptor Antagonist

3. Antiparkinson Agent

4. Anticholinergic

5. Dopamine Agonist

6. Anticonvulsant

7. Analgesics (Opioid and Nonopioid)

8. Skeletal Muscle Relaxant

9. Benzodiazepines

10. Serotonin Receptor Agonist

Alzheimer Disease

GENERIC	BRAND	CLASS
Donepezil	Aricept	Central Cholinesterase Inhibitor
Memantine	Namenda	N-methyl-D-aspartate (NMDA) Receptor Antagonist

Parkinson Disease

GENERIC	BRAND	CLASS
Carbidopa + Levodopa	Sinemet	Antiparkinson Agent
Benztropine	Cogentin	Anticholinergic
Pramipexole	Mirapex	Dopamine Agonist
Ropinirole	Requip	Dopamine Agonist

Seizure

CLASS: Anticonvulsant	
GENERIC	BRAND
Primidone	Mysoline
Phenytoin	Dilantin
Carbamazepine	Tegretol
Divalproex	Depakote, Depakote ER
Gabapentin	Neurontin
Lamotrigine	Lamictal
Levetiracetam	Keppra
Oxcarbazepine	Trileptal
Pregabalin	Lyrica
Topiramate	Topamax

Anxiety

CLASS: Benzodiazepines	
GENERIC	**BRAND**
Clonazepam	Klonopin
Alprazolam	Xanax
Buspirone	Buspar
Lorazepam	Ativan
Diazepam	Valium

Muscle Spasm

CLASS: Skeletal Muscle Relaxant	
GENERIC	**BRAND**
Baclofen	Lioresal
Carisoprodol	Soma
Cyclobenzaprine	Flexeril
Methocarbamol	Robaxin

Pain Management

CLASS: Nonopioid Analgesics	
GENERIC	**BRAND**
Aspirin	Ecotrin
Acetaminophen	Tylenol
Diclofenac Sodium	Voltaren, Cambia, Zipsor, Zorvolex
Ibuprofen	Motrin, Advil
Naproxen	Anaprox
Ketorolac	Toradol
Celecoxib	Celebrex
Indomethacin	Indocin, Tivorbex
Meloxicam	Mobic
Lidocaine Patch	Lidoderm

| CLASS: Opioid Analgesics ||
GENERIC	BRAND
Morphine Sulfate	MS Contin, Avinza, Kadian
Hydromorphone	Dilaudid
Hydrocodone Bitartrate	Zohydro ER, Hysingla ER, Vantrela ER
Hydrocodone + Acetaminophen	Norco, Vicodin, Lorcet
Oxycodone	OxyContin
Fentanyl	Duragesic Patch, Lonsys
Tramadol	Ultram
Buprenorphine + Naloxone	Suboxone, Bunavail, Zubsolv
Acetaminophen + Butalbital	Phrenilin Forte, Phrenilin, Bupap, Orbivan CF

Migraine Headaches

| CLASS: Serotonin Receptor Agonist ||
GENERIC	BRAND
Rizatriptan	Maxalt
Sumatriptan	Imitrex

| CLASS: Alpha 2 Adrenergic Agonist ||
GENERIC	BRAND
Tizanidine	Zanaflex

10.

◦◦⌒◦◦

NUTRITIONAL

This chapter covers Nutritional supplementation, Congestion, Nasal Dryness, and Dental Carries Prevention. The pharmacologic classes used are: Vitamins, Electrolyte, Decongestant, and Oral Rinse.

Nutritional Supplementation

CLASS: Vitamins	
GENERIC	**BRAND**
Calcium	Tums, Oysco
Calcium + Cholecalciferol	Os-Cal Ultra, Caltrate 600 + D3
Ergocalciferol	Vitamin D2
Calcitriol	Rocaltrol

CLASS: Electrolyte	
GENERIC	**BRAND**
Magnesium Oxide	Mag-Ox 400
Potassium Chloride	Klor-Con

Congestion, Nasal Dryness

CLASS: Decongestant	
GENERIC	BRAND
Sodium Chloride	Ocean, Ayr Saline

Dental Caries Prevention

CLASS: Oral Rinse	
GENERIC	BRAND
Sodium Fluoride	PreviDent

11.

ONCOLOGIC

This chapter only has Breast Cancer and the pharmacologic class used here is Antineoplastic.

Breast Cancer

CLASS: Antineoplastic	
GENERIC	**BRAND**
Tamoxifen	Soltamox
Anastrozole	Arimidex

12.

⟨∽⟩

OPHTHALMOLOGIC

The disease states covered in this chapter are: Glaucoma, Allergic Conjunctivitis, Infection, Bacterial Conjunctivitis, and Corneal Ulcer. The pharmacologic classes used are: Antiglaucoma, Antihistamine, and Antibiotic.

Glaucoma

CLASS: Antiglaucoma	
GENERIC	**BRAND**
Brimonidine tartrate	Alphagan P
Bimatoprost	Lumigan
Latanoprost	Xalatan
Travoprost	Travatan Z
Timolol	Timoptic
Dorzolamide	Trusopt
Dorzolamide + Timolol	Cosopt

Allergic Conjunctivitis

CLASS: Antihistamine	
GENERIC	**BRAND**
Olopatadine	Patanol, Pataday
Naphazoline + Pheniramine	Naphcon-A, Opcon-A

Infection, Bacterial Conjunctivitis, Corneal Ulcer

CLASS: Antibiotic	
GENERIC	BRAND
Ofloxacin	Ocuflox

13.

⁓

PSYCHIATRIC

This chapter covers the following disease states:

1. Attention-deficit hyperactivity disorder (ADHD)

2. Anxiety

3. Depression

4. Schizophrenia

5. Bipolar

6. Psychosis

7. Narcolepsy

8. Insomnia

9. Obesity

The pharmacologic classes used are:

1. Antidepressant

2. Antipsychotic

3. CNS Stimulant

4. Sedative

5. Appetite Suppressant

Attention-deficit hyperactivity disorder (ADHD), Narcolepsy

CLASS: CNS Stimulant	
GENERIC	**BRAND**
Atomoxetine	Strattera
Dexmethylphenidate Hydrochloride	Focalin
Dextroamphetamine + Amphetamine	Adderall
Lisdexamfetamine	Vyvanse
Methylphenidate	Ritalin, Concerta

Depression, Anxiety

CLASS: Antidepressant		
GENERIC	**BRAND**	**SUBCLASS**
Citalopram	Celexa	Selective Serotonin Reuptake Inhibitor (SSRI)
Escitalopram	Lexapro	SSRI
Fluoxetine	Prozac	SSRI
Paroxetine	Paxil	SSRI
Sertraline	Zoloft	SSRI
Venlafaxine	Effexor	Serotonin/Norepinephrine Reuptake Inhibitor (SNRI)
Desvenlafaxine	Pristiq	SNRI
Duloxetine	Cymbalta	SNRI
Amitriptyline	Elavil	Tricyclic Antidepressant (TCA)
Nortriptyline	Pamelor	TCA
Doxepin	Sinequan, Silenor	TCA
Mirtazapine	Remeron	Serotonin and α_2-adrenergic Antagonist
Trazodone	Desyrel	Antidepressant, Histamine and alpha1-adrenergic receptor antagonist
Vilazodone	Viibryd	Antidepressant, Mixed serotonergic effects
Bupropion	Wellbutrin, Zyban	Dopamine and Norepinephrine Reuptake Inhibitor, Smoking Cessation Aids

Schizophrenia, Bipolar, Psychosis

CLASS: Antipsychotic	
GENERIC	**BRAND**
Haloperidol	Haldol
Aripiprazole	Abilify
Lurasidone	Latuda
Olanzapine	Zyprexa
Quetiapine	Seroquel
Risperidone	Risperdal
Ziprasidone	Geodon
Lithium	Lithobid, Eskalith

Insomnia

CLASS: Sedative	
GENERIC	**BRAND**
Eszopiclone	Lunesta
Temazepam	Restoril
Triazolam	Halcion
Zolpidem	Ambien

Obesity Management

CLASS: CNS stimulant (Appetite Suppressant)	
GENERIC	**BRAND**
Phentermine	Adipex-P, Lomaira

14.

RESPIRATORY

The disease states covered in this chapter are: Asthma, COPD, and Allergic Rhinitis. The pharmacologic classes used are: Beta-2 Agonist, Corticosteroid, Leukotriene Modifiers, and Antihistamines.

Asthma and COPD

CLASS: Beta-2 Agonists	
GENERIC	**BRAND**
Albuterol	Proair HFA, Proventil HFA, Ventolin HFA
Ipratropium Bromide	Atrovent HFA
Albuterol + Ipratropium	Combivent Respimat, DuoNeb
Tiotropium	Spiriva Handihaler

CLASS: Corticosteroid	
GENERIC	**BRAND**
Prednisone	Deltasone
Prednisolone Oral	Orapred, Prelone
Methylprednisolone	Medrol
Beclomethasone Dipropionate	Qvar
Budesonide	Pulmicort Flexhaler
Fluticasone furoate	Arnuity Ellipta
Fluticasone + Salmeterol	Advair HFA, Advair Diskus
Mometasone + Formoterol	Dulera
Budesonide + Formoterol	Symbicort

CLASS: Leukotriene Modifiers	
GENERIC	BRAND
Montelukast	Singulair

Allergic Rhinitis

CLASS: Antihistamines	
GENERIC	BRAND
Diphenhydramine	Benadryl
Loratadine	Claritin, Alavert
Cetirizine	Zyrtec
Fexofenadine	Allegra
Levocetirizine	Xyzal
Hydroxyzine	Atarax, Vistaril
Azelastine (Nasal)	Astelin, Astepro

CLASS: Corticosteroid	
GENERIC	BRAND
Fluticasone	Flonase, Veramyst
Mometasone Nasal	Nasonex
Triamcinolone	Nasacort

15.

❦

UROLOGIC

The disease states covered here are:

1. Benign Prostate Hyperplasia
2. Overactive Bladder (or Urinary Incontinence)
3. Erectile Dysfunction
4. Testosterone Deficiency, and
5. Hypogonadism.

The pharmacologic classes used are:

1. Alpha Adrenergic Antagonists
2. 5 Alpha Reductase Inhibitors
3. Anticholinergic agents
4. Beta 3 Agonist
5. Phosphodiesterase inhibitor, and
6. Testosterone supplements.

Benign Prostatic Hyperplasia

| CLASS: Alpha Adrenergic Antagonists ||
GENERIC	BRAND
Alfuzosin	Uroxatral
Doxazosin	Cardura
Prazosin (only used for hypertension)	Minipress, Prazo, Prazin

Terazosin	Hytrin
Tamsulosin	Flomax

CLASS: 5 Alpha Reductase Inhibitors	
GENERIC	**BRAND**
Dutasteride	Avodart
Finasteride	Proscar, Propecia

Overactive Bladder (Urinary Incontinence)

CLASS: Anticholinergic agents	
GENERIC	**BRAND**
Oxybutynin	Ditropan
Solifenacin	Vesicare
Tolterodine	Detrol LA

CLASS: Beta 3 Agonist	
GENERIC	**BRAND**
Mirabegron	Myrbetriq

Erectile Dysfunction

CLASS: Phosphodiesterase inhibitor	
GENERIC	**BRAND**
Sildenafil	Viagra, Revatio
Tadalafil	Cialis

Testosterone Deficiency, Hypogonadism

CLASS: Testosterone supplements	
GENERIC	**BRAND**
Testosterone	Androgel, Androderm

PART 2

GENERIC NAMES

16.

~~~

ALPHABETICAL ORDER
BY GENERIC

#	GENERIC	BRAND	CLASS	INDICATION
1	Acetaminophen	Tylenol	Analgesic	Pain
2	Acetaminophen + Butalbital	Phrenilin Forte, Phrenilin, Bupap, Orbivan CF	Analgesic + Barbiturate Combo	Pain
3	Acetaminophen + Hydrocodone	Norco, Vicodin, Lorcet	Analgesic (Narcotic)	Pain
4	Acyclovir	Zovirax	Antiviral	Infection
5	Adalimumab	Humira	DMARD, Antipsoriatic	Rheumatoid Arthritis, Psoriatic Arthritis, Crohn Disease, Ulcerative Colitis
6	Albuterol	Proair HFA, Proventil HFA, Ventolin HFA	Bronchodilator	Asthma
7	Albuterol Sulfate + Ipratropium Bromide	Combivent Respimat	Respiratory Inhalant Combo	Chronic Obstructive Pulmonary Disease (COPD)
8	Alendronate	Fosamax	Bisphosphonate	Osteoporosis

#	GENERIC	BRAND	CLASS	INDICATION
9	Alfuzosin	Uroxatral	Alpha Blocker	Benign Prostate Hyperplasia (BPH), Hypertension
10	Allopurinol	Zyloprim	Xanthine Oxidase Inhibitor	Gout
11	Alprazolam	Xanax	Benzodiazepines, Antianxiety, Anxiolytic	Anxiety
12	Amiodarone	Cordarone	Antiarrhythmic	Arrhythmias
13	Amitriptyline	Elavil	Antidepressant (Tricyclic)	Depression
14	Amlodipine	Norvasc	Calcium Channel Blocker	Hypertension
15	Amlodipine + Benazepril	Lotrel	Calcium Channel Blocker + Angiotensin-converting enzyme (ACE) Inhibitor	Hypertension
16	Amoxicillin	Amoxil	Antibiotic	Infection
17	Amoxicillin + Clavulanate	Augmentin	Antibiotic	Infection
18	Anastrozole	Arimidex	Antineoplastic, Aromatase Inhibitor	Breast Cancer
19	Apixaban	Eliquis	Anticoagulant	Stroke, Deep Vein Thrombosis, Pulmonary Embolism
20	Aripiprazole	Abilify	Antipsychotic, Antimanic	Schizophrenia, Bipolar, Psychosis, Depression
21	Aspirin	Ecotrin	Antiplatelet, NSAID, Salicylate	Pain, Fever, Stroke, Acute Coronary Syndrome
22	Atenolol	Tenormin	Beta Blocker	Hypertension
23	Atenolol + Chlorthalidone	Tenoretic	Beta Blocker + Diuretic	Hypertension, Edema

#	GENERIC	BRAND	CLASS	INDICATION
24	Atomoxetine	Strattera	CNS Stimulant	Attention-deficit hyperactivity disorder (ADHD), Narcolepsy
25	Atorvastatin	Lipitor	Antihyperlipidemic, HMG-CoA Reductase Inhibitor	Cholesterol
26	Azelastine	Astelin, Astepro	Antihistamine	Allergic Rhinitis
27	Azithromycin	Z-Pak, Zithromax	Antibiotic (Macrolide)	Infection
28	Bacitracin + Neomycin + Polymyxin B	Neosporin	Antibiotic	Infection
29	Baclofen	Lioresal	Skeletal Muscle Relaxant	Muscle Relaxer
30	Beclomethasone Dipropionate	Qvar	Corticosteroid	Asthma
31	Benazepril	Lotensin	Angiotensin-converting enzyme (ACE) Inhibitor	Hypertension
32	Benzonatate	Tessalon Perles	Antitussive	Cough
33	Benztropine	Cogentin	Antiparkinson Agent, Anticholinergic	Parkinson Disease
34	Betamethasone Dipropionate + Clotrimazole	Lotrisone	Corticosteroid, Antifungal	Tinea Cruris, Tinea Corporis, Tinea Pedis
35	Bimatoprost	Lumigan	Antiglaucoma	Glaucoma
36	Bisoprolol	Zebeta	Beta Blocker	Hypertension
37	Brimonidine tartrate	Alphagan P	Alpha Blocker	Glaucoma
38	Budesonide	Pulmicort Flexhaler	Corticosteroid	Asthma
39	Budesonide + Formoterol	Symbicort	Respiratory Inhalant Combo	Asthma, Chronic Obstructive Pulmonary Disease (COPD)

#	GENERIC	BRAND	CLASS	INDICATION
40	Bumetanide	Bumex, Burinex	Diuretic (Loop)	Edema, Hypertension
41	Buprenorphine + Naloxone	Suboxone, Bunavail, Zubsolv	Opioid partial agonist and antagonist combination	Opioid Dependence
42	Bupropion	Wellbutrin, Zyban	Antidepressant, Smoking Cessation Aids	Depression, Smoking Cessation
43	Buspirone	Buspar	Benzodiazepines, Antianxiety, Anxiolytic	Anxiety, Smoking Cessation
44	Calcitriol	Rocaltrol	Vitamin D Analogs	Calcium Deficiency with Hypoparathyroidism
45	Calcium	Tums, Oysco	Antacid	Calcium Supplementation, Heart burn
46	Calcium + Cholecalciferol	Os-Cal Ultra, Caltrate 600 + D3	Vitamins, Fat-Soluble	Calcium Supplementation
47	Canagliflozin	Invokana	Sodium-glucose cotransporter 2 inhibitor	Diabetes
48	Carbamazepine	Tegretol	Anticonvulsant	Seizure, Bipolar disorder
49	Carbidopa + Levodopa	Sinemet, Sinemet CR	Antiparkinson Agent	Parkinson Disease
50	Carisoprodol	Soma	Skeletal Muscle Relaxant	Muscle Relaxer
51	Carvedilol	Coreg	Beta Blocker	Hypertension
52	Cefdinir	Omnicef	Antibiotic	Infection
53	Celecoxib	Celebrex	Nonsteroidal anti-inflammatory drugs (NSAID)	Pain
54	Cephalexin	Keflex	Antibiotic	Infection
55	Cetirizine	Zyrtec	Antihistamine	Allergy, Hay Fever, Urticaria

#	GENERIC	BRAND	CLASS	INDICATION
56	Chlorhexidine	Peridex, PerioGard, PerioChip	Antibiotic	Antibacterial Cleansing Agent
57	Chlorthalidone	Hygroton, Thalitone	Diuretic (Thiazide)	Edema, Hypertension, Heart Failure
58	Ciprofloxacin Oral	Cipro	Antibiotic (Fluoroquinolone)	Infection
59	Citalopram	Celexa	Antidepressant, SSRI	Depression
60	Clindamycin	Cleocin	Antibiotic	Infection
61	Clobetasol	Impoyz, Temovate	Corticosteroid	Psoriasis
62	Clonazepam	Klonopin	Benzodiazepines	Anxiety
63	Clonidine	Catapres	α2-Adrenergic Agonist	Hypertension
64	Clopidogrel	Plavix	Antiplatelet	Stroke, Acute Coronary Syndrome
65	Colchicine	Colcrys	Uricosuric Agent	Gout
66	Conjugated Estrogens + Medroxyprogesterone	Prempro	Hormone Replacement	Menopause
67	Cyanocobalamin	Vitamin B12	Vitamins, Water-Soluble	Nutritional Supplementation
68	Cyclobenzaprine	Flexeril	Skeletal Muscle Relaxant	Muscle Relaxer
69	Cyclosporine	Neoral, Sandimmune, Gengraf	Immunosuppressant, DMARD, Calcineurin Inhibitor	Solid Organ Transplantation, Rheumatoid Arthritis, Psoriasis
70	Dapagliflozin	Farxiga	Sodium-glucose cotransporter 2 inhibitor	Diabetes
71	Desogestrel + Ethinyl Estradiol	Apri, Cyclessa, Enskyce, Viorele	Contraceptive	Birth Control
72	Desvenlafaxine	Pristiq	Serotonin/ Norepinephrine Reuptake Inhibitor	Depression

#	GENERIC	BRAND	CLASS	INDICATION
73	Dexlansoprazole	Dexilant	Proton Pump Inhibitor	Gastroesophageal Reflux Disease (GERD)
74	Dexmethylphenidate Hydrochloride	Focalin	CNS Stimulant	Attention-deficit hyperactivity disorder (ADHD), Narcolepsy
75	Dextroamphetamine + Amphetamine	Adderall	CNS Stimulant	Attention-deficit hyperactivity disorder (ADHD), Narcolepsy
76	Diazepam	Valium	Benzodiazepines, Sedative	Anxiety, Sleep, Muscle Relaxer
77	Diclofenac Sodium	Voltaren, Cambia, Zipsor, Zorvolex	Nonsteroidal anti-inflammatory drugs (NSAID)	Pain, Osteoarthritis, Rheumatoid Arthritis
78	Dicyclomine	Bentyl	Anticholinergic	Irritable Bowel Sndrome (IBS) / Abdominal Cramps
79	Digoxin	Lanoxin	Antiarrhythmic	Heart Failure, Arrhythmia, Atrial fibrillation
80	Diltiazem	Cardizem, Cartia XT	Calcium Channel Blocker	Hypertension, Antiarrhythmic, Angina
81	Diphenhydramine	Benadryl	Antihistamine, Antiemetic	Allergic Reaction, Insomnia, Cough, Motion Sickness
82	Divalproex	Depakote, Depakote ER	Anticonvulsant	Seizure, Bipolar disorder, Mania, Migraine Prophylaxis
83	Docusate Sodium	Colace	Laxative	Constipation
84	Donepezil	Aricept	Central Cholinesterase Inhibitor	Alzheimer Disease
85	Dorzolamide	Trusopt	Antiglaucoma	Glaucoma, Ocular Hypertension
86	Dorzolamide + Timolol	Cosopt	Antiglaucoma	Glaucoma, Ocular Hypertension

#	GENERIC	BRAND	CLASS	INDICATION
87	Doxazosin	Cardura, Cardura-XL	Alpha Blocker	Benign Prostate Hyperplasia (BPH), Hypertension
88	Doxepin	Sinequan, Silenor	Antidepressant (Tricyclic)	Depression, Anxiety, Insomnia
89	Doxycycline	Vibramycin	Antibiotic (Tetracycline)	Infection
90	Drospirenone + Ethinyl estradiol	Yaz	Contraceptive	Birth Control
91	Dulaglutide	Trulicity	Glucagon-Like Peptide-1 Receptor Agonist	Diabetes
92	Duloxetine	Cymbalta	Serotonin/Norepinephrine Reuptake Inhibitor	Depression
93	Dutasteride	Avodart	5-Alpha-Reductase Inhibitor	Benign Prostate Hyperplasia (BPH)
94	Empagliflozin	Jardiance	Antidiabetic, SGLT2 Inhibitor	Diabetes
95	Emtricitabine	Emtriva	HIV, NRTI	HIV Infection
96	Enalapril	Vasotec	Angiotensin-converting enzyme (ACE) Inhibitor	Hypertension
97	Enoxaparin	Lovenox	Anticoagulant	Stroke, Deep Vein Thrombosis, Angina, Acute Coronary Syndromes
98	Epinephrine Auto-Injector	Drenaclick, Auvi-Q, EpiPen, EpiPen Jr	Anaphylaxis Agent	Heart Attack, Hypotension Associated with Septic Shock, Anaphylaxis
99	Ergocalciferol	Vitamin D	Vitamins, Fat-Soluble	Nutritional Supplementation
100	Erythromycin	Erythrocin	Antibiotic (Macrolide)	Infection
101	Escitalopram	Lexapro	Antidepressant, SSRI	Depression

#	GENERIC	BRAND	CLASS	INDICATION
102	Esomeprazole	Nexium	Proton Pump Inhibitor	Gastroesophageal Reflux Disease (GERD), Ulcers, Erosive Esophagitis
103	Estradiol oral	Estrace	Estrogen Derivatives	Osteoporosis, Breast Cancer, Prostate Cancer
104	Estrogens, Conjugated	Premarin	Estrogen Derivatives	Menopause, Female Hypogonadism, Osteoporosis, Prostate Cancer, Abnormal Uterine Bleeding
105	Eszopiclone	Lunesta	Sedative	Insomnia
106	Ethinyl Estradiol + Etonogestrel	NuvaRing	Contraceptive	Birth Control
107	Ethinyl Estradiol + Levonorgestrel	Twirla	Contraceptive	Birth Control
108	Ethinyl Estradiol + Norethindrone	Necon 777	Contraceptive	Birth Control
109	Ethinyl Estradiol + Norgestimate	Trinessa-28, Ortho Tri-Cyclen, Ortho Tri-Cyclen Lo	Contraceptive	Birth Control
110	Ethinyl Estradiol + Norgestrel	Cryselle	Contraceptive	Birth Control
111	Exenatide	Byetta, Bydureon	Glucagon-Like Peptide-1 Receptor Agonist	Diabetes
112	Ezetimibe	Zetia	Antihyperlipidemic	Cholesterol
113	Ezetimibe + Simvastatin	Vytorin	Antihyperlipidemic	Cholesterol
114	Famotidine	Pepcid	Histamine H2 Antagonist	Heartburn
115	Fenofibrate	Tricor, Trilipix, Antara, Fenoglide, Lipofen, Lofibra, Trilipix	Antihyperlipidemic, Fibric Acid Derivative	Cholesterol

#	GENERIC	BRAND	CLASS	INDICATION
116	Fentanyl	Duragesic Patch, Lonsys	Analgesic (Opioid)	Pain
117	Ferrous Sulfate	Feosol, Fer-In-Sol	Iron Product	Anemia
118	Fexofenadine	Allegra	Antihistamine	Allergic Rhinitis, Urticaria
119	Finasteride	Proscar, Propecia	5-Alpha-Reductase Inhibitor	Benign Prostate Hyperplasia (BPH)
120	Flecainide	Tambacor	Antiarrhythmic	Arrhythmias
121	Fluconazole	Diflucan	Antifungal	Infection
122	Fluoxetine	Prozac	Antidepressant, SSRI	Depression, Anxiety
123	Fluticasone	Flonase, Veramyst, Flovent HFA, Arnuity Ellipta, Flovent Diskus	Intranasal Adrenal Glucocorticosteroid	Asthma, Allergic Rhinitis, Nasal Polyps
124	Fluticasone + Salmeterol	Advair Diskus, Advair HFA	Corticosteroid + Beta Blocker	Asthma
125	Folic Acid	Folate, Folvite	Vitamins, Water-Soluble	Nutritional Supplementation
126	Formoterol + Mometasone	Dulera	Respiratory Inhalant Combos, Bronchodilator	Asthma
127	Furosemide	Lasix	Diuretic (Loop)	Edema, Hypertension, Hyperkalemia
128	Gabapentin	Neurontin	Anticonvulsant	Seizure, Neuralgia
129	Gemfibrozil	Lopid	Antihyperlipidemic, Fibric Acid Derivative	Cholesterol, Triglyceride
130	Glimepiride	Amaryl	Antidiabetic, Sulfonylureas	Diabetes
131	Glipizide	Glucotrol	Antidiabetic, Sulfonylureas	Diabetes

#	GENERIC	BRAND	CLASS	INDICATION
132	Glyburide	Micronase, Diabeta	Antidiabetic, Sulfonylureas	Diabetes
133	Guaifenesin	Mucinex	Expectorant	Cough
134	Guaifenesin + Pseudoephedrine + Codeine	Cheratussin DAC, Virtussin DAC	Antitussive, Narcotic	Cough with Congestion
135	Guanfacine	Intuniv	α2-Adrenergic Agonist	Hypertension
136	Haloperidol	Haldol	Antipsychotic	Schizophrenia, Psychosis
137	HCTZ + Losartan	Hyzaar	Diuretic + Angiotensin II Receptor Blocker	Hypertension, Edema
138	HCTZ + Olmesartan	Benicar HCT	Diuretic + Angiotensin II Receptor Blocker	Hypertension, Edema
139	HCTZ + Triamterene	Dyazide, Maxzide	Diuretic (Potassium-sparing and Thiazide)	Hypertension, Edema
140	HCTZ + Valsartan	Diovan HCT	Diuretic + Angiotensin II Receptor Blocker	Hypertension, Edema
141	Hydralazine	Apresoline	Peripheral Vasodilator	Hypertension
142	Hydrochlorothiazide (HCTZ)	Microzide	Diuretic (Thiazide)	Edema, Hypertension
143	Hydrochlorothiazide (HCTZ) + Lisinopril	Zestoretic	Diuretic + Angiotensin-converting enzyme (ACE) Inhibitor	Hypertension, Edema
144	Hydrocodone Bitartrate	Zohydro ER, Hysingla ER, Vantrela ER	Analgesic (Opioid)	Pain
145	Hydrocortisone Topical	Cortisone	Corticosteroid	Inflammation
146	Hydromorphone	Dilaudid	Analgesic (Opioid)	Pain

#	GENERIC	BRAND	CLASS	INDICATION
147	Hydroxychloroquine	Plaquenil	Aminoquinoline	Lupus, Rheumatoid Arthritis, Malaria
148	Hydroxyzine	Atarax, Vistaril	Antihistamine, Antiemetic	Anxiety, Sedation, Pruritus
149	Ibuprofen	Motrin, Advil	Nonsteroidal anti-inflammatory drugs (NSAID)	Pain, Fever, Inflammation
150	Indomethacin	Indocin, Tivorbex	Nonsteroidal anti-inflammatory drugs (NSAID)	Pain, Inflammation, Acute Gouty Arthritis
151	Insulin Aspart	Novolog	Antidiabetic, Insulin, Rapid Acting	Diabetes
152	Insulin Degludec	Tresiba	Antidiabetic, Insulin, Long Acting	Diabetes
153	Insulin Detemir	Levemir	Antidiabetic, Insulin, Long Acting	Diabetes
154	Insulin Glargine	Lantus	Antidiabetic, Insulin, Long Acting	Diabetes
155	Insulin Human	Humulin R, Novolin R	Antidiabetic, Insulin, Short Acting	Diabetes
156	Insulin Lispro	Humalog	Antidiabetic, Insulin, Rapid Acting	Diabetes
157	Ipratropium Bromide	Atrovent HFA	Bronchodilator	Chronic Obstructive Pulmonary Disease (COPD)
158	Irbesartan	Avapro	Angiotensin II Receptor Blocker	Hypertension
159	Isosorbide Mononitrate	Imdur	Nitrate	Angina
160	Ketoconazole Topical	Nizoral	Antifungal	Infection

#	GENERIC	BRAND	CLASS	INDICATION
161	Ketorolac	Toradol	Nonsteroidal anti-inflammatory drugs (NSAID)	Pain
162	Labetalol	Normodyne	Beta Blocker	Hypertension
163	Lamotrigine	Lamictal	Anticonvulsant	Seizure, Bipolar disorder
164	Lansoprazole	Prevacid	Proton Pump Inhibitor	Gastroesophageal Reflux Disease (GERD), Ulcers, Erosive Esophagitis
165	Latanoprost	Xalatan	Prostaglandin	Glaucoma
166	Levetiracetam	Keppra	Anticonvulsant	Seizure
167	Levocetirizine	Xyzal	Antihistamine	Allergic Rhinitis, Urticaria
168	Levofloxacin	Levaquin	Antibiotic (Fluoroquinolone)	Infection
169	Levothyroxine	Synthroid	Thyroid	Hypothyroidism
170	Lidocaine Patch	Lidoderm	Local Anesthetic	Pain
171	Linaclotide	Linzess	Gastrointestinal, IBS Agent	Irritable Bowel Syndrome, Chronic Idiopathic Constipation
172	Linagliptin	Tradjenta	Dipeptidyl Peptidase 4 Inhibitor	Diabetes
173	Liothyronine	Cytomel, Triostat	Thyroid	Hypothyroidism
174	Liraglutide	Victoza, Saxenda	Glucagon-Like Peptide-1 Receptor Agonist	Diabetes
175	Lisdexamfetamine	Vyvanse	CNS stimulant	Attention-deficit hyperactivity disorder (ADHD), Narcolepsy
176	Lisinopril	Prinivil, Zestril	Angiotensin-converting enzyme (ACE) Inhibitor	Hypertension

#	GENERIC	BRAND	CLASS	INDICATION
177	Lithium	Lithobid, Eskalith	Antimanic	Bipolar Disorder
178	Loratadine	Claritin, Alavert	Antihistamine	Allergic Rhinitis, Urticaria
179	Lorazepam	Ativan	Benzodiazepines, Antianxiety, Anxiolytic, Sedative, Anticonvulsant	Anxiety, Sleep, Seizure
180	Losartan	Cozaar	Angiotensin II Receptor Blocker	Hypertension
181	Lovastatin	Mevacor, Altoprev	Antihyperlipidemic, HMG-CoA Reductase Inhibitor	Cholesterol
182	Lurasidone	Latuda	Antipsychotic	Schizophrenia, Bipolar, Psychosis
183	Magnesium Oxide	Mag-Ox 400	Antacid, Electrolyte	Antacid, Magnesium Supplementation
184	Meclizine	Antivert, Bonine, Dramamine	Antihistamine, Antiemetic	Motion Sickness, Vertigo
185	Medroxyprogesterone	Provera, Depo-Provera	Progestin hormone	Abnormal Uterine Bleeding, Contraception
186	Meloxicam	Mobic	Nonsteroidal anti-inflammatory drugs (NSAID)	Osteoarthritis
187	Memantine	Namenda	NMDA Antagonist	Alzheimer Disease, Dementia
188	Menthol	Bengay Cold Therapy, Icy Hot Naturals	Analgesic	Pain
189	Mesalamine	Asacol	5-Aminosalicylic Acid Derivatives	Ulcerative Colitis
190	Metformin	Glucophage	Biguanide	Diabetes
191	Metformin + Sitagliptin	Janumet XR	Antidiabetic, Biguanides + Dipeptyl Peptidase-IV Inhibitor	Diabetes

#	GENERIC	BRAND	CLASS	INDICATION
192	Methimazole	Tapazole	Thyroid	Hyperthyroidism, Graves Disease
193	Methocarbamol	Robaxin	Skeletal Muscle Relaxant	Muscle Relaxer
194	Methotrexate	Trexall	Immunosuppressant, Antineoplstic, DMARD	Rheumatoid Arthritis, Psoriasis, Cancer, Neoplasms, Leukemia
195	Methylcellulose	Citrucel	Laxative	Constipation
196	Methylphenidate	Ritalin, Concerta	CNS Stimulant	Attention-deficit hyperactivity disorder (ADHD), Narcolepsy
197	Methylprednisolone	Medrol	Corticosteroid, Anti-inflammatory	Inflammation, Allergic Condition
198	Metoclopramide	Reglan	Antiemetic, Prokinetic	Nausea and Vomiting, Diabetic Gastroparesis, GERD
199	Metoprolol	Toprol XL, Lopressor	Beta Blocker	Hypertension
200	Metronidazole	Flagyl	Antifungal, Bacterial vaginosis, Intestinal infections	Infection
201	Minocycline	Dynacin, Minocin, Solodyn	Antibiotic (Tetracycline)	Infection
202	Mirabegron	Myrbetriq	Beta 3 Agonist	Overactive Bladder
203	Mirtazapine	Remeron	Antidepressant, Serotonin and α_2-adrenergic Antagonist	Depression
204	Mometasone Nasal	Nasonex	Corticosteroid	Allergic Rhinitis
205	Montelukast	Singulair	Leukotriene Inhibitor	Asthma, Bronchospasm, Allergic Rhinitis
206	Morphine Sulfate	MS Contin, Avinza, Kadian	Analgesic (Opioid)	Pain

#	GENERIC	BRAND	CLASS	INDICATION
207	Mupirocin	Bactroban	Antibiotic	Infection
208	Mycophenolate	CellCept, Myfortic	Immunosuppressant	Transplant (Heart, Liver, Kidney)
209	Naphazoline + Pheniramine	Naphcon-A, Opcon-A, Visine-A	Antihistamine + Decongestant	Allergic Conjunctivitis
210	Naproxen	Anaprox	Nonsteroidal anti-inflammatory drugs (NSAID)	Pain, Inflammation
211	Nebivolol	Bystolic	Beta Blocker	Hypertension
212	Niacin	Niaspan, Slo-Niacin	Antihyperlipidemic	Cholesterol
213	Nifedipine	Procardia, Adalat	Calcium Channel Blocker	Hypertension
214	Nitrofurantoin	Macrobid, Macrodantin	Antibiotic	Infection
215	Nitroglycerin	Nitrostat, Minitran	Nitrate, Vasodilator	Angina
216	Norethindrone	Errin, Heather, Camila	Contraceptive	Birth Control
217	Nortriptyline	Pamelor	Antidepressant (Tricyclic)	Depression
218	Nystatin	Mycostatin, Nyamyc, Nystop	Antifungal	Infection
219	Ofloxacin	Ocuflox	Antibiotic (Quinolone)	Infection, Bacterial Conjunctivitis, Corneal Ulcer
220	Olanzapine	Zyprexa	Antipsychotic, Antimanic	Schizophrenia, Bipolar, Psychosis
221	Olmesartan	Benicar	Angiotensin II Receptor Blocker	Hypertension
222	Olopatadine	Patanol, Pataday	Antihistamine	Allergic Conjunctivitis
223	Omega-3 Fatty Acid Ethyl Esters	Lovaza	Antihyperlipidemic	High Triglyceride

#	GENERIC	BRAND	CLASS	INDICATION
224	Omeprazole	Prilosec	Proton Pump Inhibitor	Gastroesophageal Reflux Disease (GERD), Ulcers
225	Ondansetron	Zofran	Antiemetic	Nausea and Vomiting
226	Oseltamivir	Tamiflu	Antiviral	Influenza A and B
227	Oxcarbazepine	Trileptal	Anticonvulsant	Seizure
228	Oxybutynin	Ditropan	Antispasmodic Agent, Urinary	Overactive Bladder
229	Oxycodone	OxyContin	Analgesic (Opioid)	Pain
230	Pancrelipase	Creon, Zenpep	Pancreatic/ Digestive Enzyme	Pancreatic Insufficiency
231	Pantoprazole	Protonix	Proton Pump Inhibitor	Gastroesophageal Reflux Disease (GERD)
232	Paroxetine	Paxil	Antidepressant, SSRI	Depression, Obsessive-Compulsive Disorder, Anxiety
233	Penicillin VK	Pen Vee K, Penicillin V	Antibiotic (Penicillin)	Infection
234	Phentermine	Adipex-P, Lomaira	CNS stimulant, appetite suppressant	Obesity Management, Appetite Suppressant
235	Phenytoin	Dilantin	Anticonvulsant	Seizure
236	Pioglitazone	Actos	Antidiabetic, Thiazolidinediones	Diabetes
237	Polyethylene Glycol 3350	Golytely, Miralax	Laxative	Constipation, Bowel Preparation
238	Potassium Chloride	Klor-Con	Electrolyte Supplements	Hypokalemia
239	Pramipexole	Mirapex	Antiparkinson Agent, Dopamine Agonist	Parkinson Disease
240	Pravastatin	Pravachol	Antihyperlipidemic, HMG-CoA Reductase Inhibitor	Cholesterol
241	Prazosin	Minipress, Prazo, Prazin	Alpha Blocker	Hypertension

#	GENERIC	BRAND	CLASS	INDICATION
242	Prednisolone Oral	Orapred, Prelone, Pediapred	Glucocorticosteroid	Rheumatoid Arthritis, Multiple Sclerosis
243	Prednisone	Deltasone	Corticosteroid	Asthma, Rheumatoid Arthritis
244	Pregabalin	Lyrica	Anticonvulsant, Analgesic	Seizure, Neuropathic Pain
245	Primidone	Mysoline	Anticonvulsant	Seizure
246	Progesterone	Prometrium	Progestin Hormone	Prevention of Endometrial Hyperplasia, Secondary Amenorrhea
247	Promethazine	Phenergan	Antihistamine, Antiemetic	Nausea and Vomiting, Motion Sickness, Sedation, Allergy
248	Propranolol	Inderal	Beta Blocker	Hypertension
249	Quetiapine	Seroquel	Antipsychotic, Antimanic	Schizophrenia, Bipolar, Psychosis, Depression
250	Quinapril	Accupril	Angiotensin-converting enzyme (ACE) Inhibitor	Hypertension
251	Rabeprazole	Aciphex	Proton Pump Inhibitor	Gastroesophageal Reflux Disease (GERD), Duodenal Ulcer
252	Ramipril	Altace	Angiotensin-converting enzyme (ACE) Inhibitor	Hypertension
253	Ranitidine	Zantac	Histamine H2 Antagonist	Gastroesophageal Reflux Disease (GERD)
254	Ranolazine	Ranexa	Antianginal, Non-nitrates	Angina
255	Risperidone	Risperdal	Antipsychotic, Antimanic	Schizophrenia, Bipolar, Psychosis

#	GENERIC	BRAND	CLASS	INDICATION
256	Rivaroxaban	Xarelto	Anticoagulant, Factor Xa Inhibitor	Stroke, Deep Vein Thrombosis, Pulmonary Embolism
257	Rizatriptan	Maxalt	Antimigraine, Serotonin Receptor Agonist	Migraine Headaches
258	Ropinirole	Requip	Antiparkinson Agent, Dopamine Agonist	Parkinson Disease, Restless Leg Syndrome
259	Rosuvastatin	Crestor	Antihyperlipidemic, HMG-CoA Reductase Inhibitor	Cholesterol
260	Sennosides	Senna, Senokot	Laxative	Constipation
261	Sertraline	Zoloft	Antidepressant, SSRI	Depression, Anxiety, Obsessive-Compulsive Disorder, PTSD
262	Sildenafil	Viagra, Revatio	Phosphodiesterase-5 (PDE-5) Enzyme Inhibitor	Erectile Dysfunction, Pulmonary Arterial Hypertension
263	Simvastatin	Zocor	Antihyperlipidemic, HMG-CoA Reductase Inhibitor	Cholesterol
264	Sitagliptin	Januvia	Antidiabetic, DPP4 Inhibitor	Diabetes
265	Sodium Chloride	Ocean, Ayr Saline	Decongestant, Intranasal	Congestion, Nasal Dryness
266	Sodium Fluoride	PreviDent	Oral Rinse	Dental Caries Prevention
267	Solifenacin	Vesicare	Anticholinergic, Genitourinary	Overactive Bladder
268	Sotalol	Betapace, Sorine	Antiarrhythmic	Arrhythmias
269	Spironolactone	Aldactone	Diuretic (Potassium-sparing)	Edema, Hypertension, Heart Failure
270	Sucralfate	Carafate	Gastrointestinal Agent	Duodenal Ulcer

#	GENERIC	BRAND	CLASS	INDICATION
271	Sulfamethoxazole + Trimethoprim	Bactrim	Antibiotic	Infection
272	Sumatriptan	Imitrex	Antimigraine, Serotonin Receptor Agonist	Migraine Headaches
273	Tadalafil	Cialis	Phosphodiesterase-5 (PDE-5) Enzyme Inhibitor	Erectile Dysfunction, Benign Prostatic Hyperplasia (BPH), Pulmonary Arterial Hypertension
274	Tamoxifen	Soltamox	Antineoplastic	Breast Cancer
275	Tamsulosin	Flomax	Alpha Blocker	Benign Prostate Hyperplasia (BPH)
276	Telmisartan	Micardis	Angiotensin II Receptor Blocker	Hypertension
277	Temazepam	Restoril	Sedative, Hypnotic	Insomnia
278	Terazosin	Hytrin	Alpha Blocker	Benign Prostate Hyperplasia (BPH), Hypertension
279	Testosterone	Androgel, Androderm	Androgens	Testosterone Deficiency, Hypogonadism
280	Thyroid	Armour Thyroid	Thyroid	Hypothyroidism
281	Timolol	Timoptic	Antiglaucoma, Beta Blocker	Ocular Hypertension
282	Tiotropium	Spiriva Handihaler	Bronchodilator	Asthma, Chronic Obstructive Pulmonary Disease (COPD)
283	Tizanidine	Zanaflex	Alpha 2 Adrenergic Agonist	Muscle Relaxer
284	Tolterodine	Detrol LA	Anticholinergic, Genitourinary	Overactive Bladder
285	Topiramate	Topamax	Anticonvulsant	Seizure, Migraine Headache
286	Torsemide	Demadex	Diuretic (Loop)	Edema, Hypertension

#	GENERIC	BRAND	CLASS	INDICATION
287	Tramadol	Ultram	Analgesic (Opioid)	Pain
288	Travoprost	Travatan Z	Antiglaucoma	Glaucoma
289	Trazodone	Desyrel	Antidepressant	Depression
290	Tretinoin	Retin A	Acne Agent	Acne
291	Triamcinolone Topical	Kenalog, Trianex, Triacet, Nasacort AQ	Corticosteroid	Inflammation
292	Triazolam	Halcion	Sedative, Hypnotic	Insomnia
293	Valacyclovir	Valtrex	Antiviral	Infection
294	Valsartan	Diovan	Angiotensin II Receptor Blocker	Hypertension
295	Venlafaxine	Effexor	Antidepressant, SNRI	Depression, Anxiety
296	Verapamil	Calan SR	Calcium Channel Blocker	Hypertension, Arrhythmia, Tachycardia
297	Vilazodone	Viibryd	Antidepressant, Mixed serotonergic effects	Depression
298	Warfarin	Coumadin	Anticoagulant	Stroke, Heart Attack, Deep Vein Thrombosis, Pulmonary Embolism
299	Ziprasidone	Geodon	Antipsychotic	Schizophrenia, Bipolar, Psychosis
300	Zolpidem	Ambien, Ambien CR, Intermezzo	Sedative, Hypnotic	Insomnia

17.

BOXED WARNING MEDS IN ALPHABETICAL ORDER BY GENERIC

B oxed warning, also known as black box warning, appears on medications that has serious or life-threatening risks.

#	GENERIC	BRAND
1	Adalimumab	Humira
2	Alprazolam	Xanax
3	Amiodarone	Cordarone
4	Amitriptyline	Elavil
5	Amlodipine + Benazepril	Lotrel
6	Amphetamine + Dextroamphetamine	Adderall
7	Apixaban	Eliquis
8	Aripiprazole	Abilify
9	Atenolol	Tenormin
10	Atomoxetine	Strattera
11	Baclofen	Lioresal
12	Benazepril	Lotensin
13	Budesonide + Formoterol	Symbicort
14	Bumetanide	Bumex, Burinex

#	GENERIC	BRAND
15	Bupropion	Wellbutrin, Zyban
16	Carbamazepine	Tegretol
17	Celecoxib	Celebrex
18	Ciprofloxacin	Cipro
19	Citalopram	Celexa
20	Clindamycin	Cleocin
21	Clonazepam	Klonopin
22	Clopidogrel	Plavix
23	Conjugated Estrogens	Premarin
24	Cyclosporine	Neoral, Sandimmune, Gengraf
25	Desvenlafaxine	Pristiq
26	Dexmethylphenidate Hydrochloride	Focalin
27	Diazepam	Valium
28	Divalproex Sodium	Depakote, Depakote ER
29	Doxepin	Sinequan, Silenor
30	Dulaglutide	Trulicity
31	Duloxetine	Cymbalta
32	Emtricitabine	Emtriva
33	Enalapril	Vasotec
34	Enoxaparin	Lovenox
35	Escitalopram	Lexapro
36	Estradiol topical	Estrace
37	Eszopiclone	Lunesta
38	Ethinyl Estradiol + Drospirenone	Yaz
39	Ethinyl Estradiol + Etonogestrel Vaginal Ring	NuvaRing
40	Ethinyl Estradiol + Norethindrone	Necon 777
41	Ethinyl Estradiol + Norgestimate	Trinessa-28, Ortho Tri-Cyclen, Ortho Tri-Cyclen Lo
42	Exenatide	Byetta, Bydureon
43	Fentanyl	Duragesic Patch, Lonsys
44	Flecainide	Tambacor
45	Fluoxetine	Prozac
46	Fluticasone + Salmeterol	Advair

#	GENERIC	BRAND
47	Furosemide	Lasix
48	Haloperidol	Haldol
49	Hydrocodone + Acetaminophen	Norco
50	Hydromorphone	Dilaudid
51	Ibuprofen	Motrin, Advil
52	Indomethacin	Indocin, Tivorbex
53	Irbesartan	Avapro
54	Ketoconazole	Nizoral
55	Ketorolac	Toradol
56	Lamotrigine	Lamictal
57	Levofloxacin	Levaquin
58	Levothyroxine	Synthroid, Levoxyl, Levothroid
59	Linaclotide	Linzess
60	Liothyronine	Cytomel
61	Liraglutide	Victoza
62	Lisdexamfetamine	Vyvanse
63	Lisinopril	Prinivil, Zestril
64	Lisinopril + HCTZ	Prinzide, Zestoretic
65	Lithium	Lithobid, Eskalith
66	Lorazepam	Ativan
67	Losartan	Cozaar
68	Losartan + HCTZ	Hyzaar
69	Lurasidone	Latuda
70	Medroxyprogesterone	Depo Provera
71	Meloxicam	Mobic
72	Metformin	Glucophage
73	Metformin + Sitagliptin	Janumet XR
74	Methotrexate	Trexall
75	Methylphenidate	Ritalin, Concerta
76	Metoclopramide	Reglan
77	Metoprolol Succinate	Toprol XL
78	Metoprolol Tartrate	Lopressor

#	GENERIC	BRAND
79	Metronidazole	Flagyl
80	Mirtazapine	Remeron
81	Montelukast	Singulair
82	Morphine	MS Contin, Avinza, Kadian
83	Mycophenolate	CellCept, Myfortic
84	Naproxen	Anaprox
85	Nortiptyline	Pamelor
86	Olanzapine	Zyprexa
87	Olmesartan	Benicar
88	Olmesartan + HCTZ	Benicar HCT
89	Oxycodone	OxyContin
90	Oxycodone + Acetaminophen	Percocet, Endocet, Roxicet
91	Paroxetine	Paxil
92	Phenytoin	Dilantin
93	Pioglitazone	Actos
94	Progesterone	Prometrium
95	Promethazine	Phenergan
96	Propranolol	Inderal
97	Quetiapine	Seroquel
98	Quinapril	Accupril
99	Ramipril	Altace
100	Rivaroxaban	Xarelto
101	Sertraline	Zoloft
102	Sotalol	Betapace, Sorine
103	Spironolactone	Aldactone
104	Tamoxifen	Soltamox
105	Telmisartan	Micardis
106	Temazepam	Restoril
107	Testosterone Gel	Androgel
108	Thyroid	Armour Thyroid
109	Ticagrelor	Brilinta
110	Tramadol	Ultram

#	GENERIC	BRAND
111	Trazodone	Desyrel
112	Triamterene + HCTZ	Dyazide, Maxzide
113	Triazolam	Halcion
114	Valsartan	Diovan
115	Valsartan + HCTZ	Diovan HCT
116	Venlafaxine	Effexor
117	Vilazodone	Viibryd
118	Warfarin	Coumadin
119	Ziprasidone	Geodon
120	Zolpidem	Ambien

PART 3

BRAND NAMES

18.

ALPHABETICAL ORDER
BY BRAND

#	BRAND	GENERIC	CLASS	INDICATION
1	Abilify	Aripiprazole	Antipsychotic, Antimanic	Schizophrenia, Bipolar, Psychosis, Depression
2	Accupril	Quinapril	Angiotensin-converting enzyme (ACE) Inhibitor	Hypertension
3	Aciphex	Rabeprazole	Proton Pump Inhibitor	Gastroesophageal Reflux Disease (GERD), Duodenal Ulcer
4	Actos	Pioglitazone	Antidiabetic, Thiazolidinediones	Diabetes
5	Adderall	Dextroamphetamine + Amphetamine	CNS Stimulant	Attention-deficit hyperactivity disorder (ADHD), Narcolepsy
6	Adipex-P, Lomaira	Phentermine	CNS stimulant, appetite suppressant	Obesity Management, Appetite Suppressant
7	Advair Diskus, Advair HFA	Fluticasone + Salmeterol	Corticosteroid + Beta Blocker	Asthma
8	Aldactone	Spironolactone	Diuretic (Potassium-sparing)	Edema, Hypertension, Heart Failure
9	Allegra	Fexofenadine	Antihistamine	Allergic Rhinitis, Urticaria
10	Alphagan P	Brimonidine tartrate	Alpha Blocker	Glaucoma

#	BRAND	GENERIC	CLASS	INDICATION
11	Altace	Ramipril	Angiotensin-converting enzyme (ACE) Inhibitor	Hypertension
12	Amaryl	Glimepiride	Antidiabetic, Sulfonylureas	Diabetes
13	Ambien, Ambien CR, Intermezzo	Zolpidem	Sedative, Hypnotic	Insomnia
14	Amoxil	Amoxicillin	Antibiotic	Infection
15	Anaprox	Naproxen	Nonsteroidal anti-inflammatory drugs (NSAID)	Pain, Inflammation
16	Androgel, Androderm	Testosterone	Androgens	Testosterone Deficiency, Hypogonadism
17	Antivert, Bonine, Dramamine	Meclizine	Antihistamine, Antiemetic	Motion Sickness, Vertigo
18	Apresoline	Hydralazine	Peripheral Vasodilator	Hypertension
19	Apri, Cyclessa, Enskyce, Viorele	Desogestrel + Ethinyl Estradiol	Contraceptive	Birth Control
20	Aricept	Donepezil	Central Cholinesterase Inhibitor	Alzheimer Disease
21	Arimidex	Anastrozole	Antineoplastic, Aromatase Inhibitor	Breast Cancer
22	Armour Thyroid	Thyroid	Thyroid	Hypothyroidism
23	Asacol	Mesalamine	5-Aminosalicylic Acid Derivatives	Ulcerative Colitis
24	Astelin, Astepro	Azelastine	Antihistamine	Allergic Rhinitis
25	Atarax, Vistaril	Hydroxyzine	Antihistamine, Antiemetic	Anxiety, Sedation, Pruritus
26	Ativan	Lorazepam	Benzodiazepines, Antianxiety, Anxiolytic, Sedative, Anticonvulsant	Anxiety, Sleep, Seizure
27	Atrovent HFA	Ipratropium Bromide	Bronchodilator	Chronic Obstructive Pulmonary Disease (COPD)
28	Augmentin	Amoxicillin + Clavulanate	Antibiotic	Infection

#	BRAND	GENERIC	CLASS	INDICATION
29	Avapro	Irbesartan	Angiotensin II Receptor Blocker	Hypertension
30	Avodart	Dutasteride	5-Alpha-Reductase Inhibitor	Benign Prostate Hyperplasia (BPH)
31	Bactrim	Sulfamethoxazole + Trimethoprim	Antibiotic	Infection
32	Bactroban	Mupirocin	Antibiotic	Infection
33	Benadryl	Diphenhydramine	Antihistamine, Antiemetic	Allergic Reaction, Insomnia, Cough, Motion Sickness
34	Bengay Cold Therapy, Icy Hot Naturals	Menthol	Analgesic	Pain
35	Benicar	Olmesartan	Angiotensin II Receptor Blocker	Hypertension
36	Benicar HCT	HCTZ + Olmesartan	Diuretic + Angiotensin II Receptor Blocker	Hypertension, Edema
37	Bentyl	Dicyclomine	Anticholinergic	Irritable Bowel Sndrome (IBS) / Abdominal Cramps
38	Betapace, Sorine	Sotalol	Antiarrhythmic	Arrhythmias
39	Bumex, Burinex	Bumetanide	Diuretic (Loop)	Edema, Hypertension
40	Buspar	Buspirone	Benzodiazepines, Antianxiety, Anxiolytic	Anxiety, Smoking Cessation
41	Byetta, Bydureon	Exenatide	Glucagon-Like Peptide-1 Receptor Agonist	Diabetes
42	Bystolic	Nebivolol	Beta Blocker	Hypertension
43	Calan SR	Verapamil	Calcium Channel Blocker	Hypertension, Arrhythmia, Tachycardia
44	Carafate	Sucralfate	Gastrointestinal Agent	Duodenal Ulcer
45	Cardizem, Cartia XT	Diltiazem	Calcium Channel Blocker	Hypertension, Antiarrhythmic, Angina
46	Cardura, Cardura-XL	Doxazosin	Alpha Blocker	Benign Prostate Hyperplasia (BPH), Hypertension
47	Catapres	Clonidine	α2-Adrenergic Agonist	Hypertension

#	BRAND	GENERIC	CLASS	INDICATION
48	Celebrex	Celecoxib	Nonsteroidal anti-inflammatory drugs (NSAID)	Pain
49	Celexa	Citalopram	Antidepressant, SSRI	Depression
50	CellCept, Myfortic	Mycophenolate	Immunosuppressant	Transplant (Heart, Liver, Kidney)
51	Cheratussin DAC, Virtussin DAC	Guaifenesin + Pseudoephedrine + Codeine	Antitussive, Narcotic	Cough with Congestion
52	Cialis	Tadalafil	Phosphodiesterase-5 (PDE-5) Enzyme Inhibitor	Erectile Dysfunction, Benign Prostatic Hyperplasia (BPH), Pulmonary Arterial Hypertension
53	Cipro	Ciprofloxacin Oral	Antibiotic (Fluoroquinolone)	Infection
54	Citrucel	Methylcellulose	Laxative	Constipation
55	Claritin, Alavert	Loratadine	Antihistamine	Allergic Rhinitis, Urticaria
56	Cleocin	Clindamycin	Antibiotic	Infection
57	Cogentin	Benztropine	Antiparkinson Agent, Anticholinergic	Parkinson Disease
58	Colace	Docusate Sodium	Laxative	Constipation
59	Colcrys	Colchicine	Uricosuric Agent	Gout
60	Combivent Respimat	Albuterol Sulfate + Ipratropium Bromide	Respiratory Inhalant Combo	Chronic Obstructive Pulmonary Disease (COPD)
61	Cordarone	Amiodarone	Antiarrhythmic	Arrhythmias
62	Coreg	Carvedilol	Beta Blocker	Hypertension
63	Cortisone	Hydrocortisone Topical	Corticosteroid	Inflammation
64	Cosopt	Dorzolamide + Timolol	Antiglaucoma	Glaucoma, Ocular Hypertension
65	Coumadin	Warfarin	Anticoagulant	Stroke, Heart Attack, Deep Vein Thrombosis, Pulmonary Embolism
66	Cozaar	Losartan	Angiotensin II Receptor Blocker	Hypertension
67	Creon, Zenpep	Pancrelipase	Pancreatic/Digestive Enzyme	Pancreatic Insufficiency

#	BRAND	GENERIC	CLASS	INDICATION
68	Crestor	Rosuvastatin	Antihyperlipidemic, HMG-CoA Reductase Inhibitor	Cholesterol
69	Cryselle	Ethinyl Estradiol + Norgestrel	Contraceptive	Birth Control
70	Cymbalta	Duloxetine	Serotonin/ Norepinephrine Reuptake Inhibitor	Depression
71	Cytomel, Triostat	Liothyronine	Thyroid	Hypothyroidism
72	Deltasone	Prednisone	Corticosteroid	Asthma, Rheumatoid Arthritis
73	Demadex	Torsemide	Diuretic (Loop)	Edema, Hypertension
74	Depakote, Depakote ER	Divalproex	Anticonvulsant	Seizure, Bipolar disorder, Mania, Migraine Prophylaxis
75	Desyrel	Trazodone	Antidepressant	Depression
76	Detrol LA	Tolterodine	Anticholinergic, Genitourinary	Overactive Bladder
77	Dexilant	Dexlansoprazole	Proton Pump Inhibitor	Gastroesophageal Reflux Disease (GERD)
78	Diflucan	Fluconazole	Antifungal	Infection
79	Dilantin	Phenytoin	Anticonvulsant	Seizure
80	Dilaudid	Hydromorphone	Analgesic (Opioid)	Pain
81	Diovan	Valsartan	Angiotensin II Receptor Blocker	Hypertension
82	Diovan HCT	HCTZ + Valsartan	Diuretic + Angiotensin II Receptor Blocker	Hypertension, Edema
83	Ditropan	Oxybutynin	Antispasmodic Agent, Urinary	Overactive Bladder
84	Drenaclick, Auvi-Q, EpiPen, EpiPen Jr	Epinephrine Auto-Injector	Anaphylaxis Agent	Heart Attack, Hypotension Associated with Septic Shock, Anaphylaxis
85	Dulera	Formoterol + Mometasone	Respiratory Inhalant Combos, Bronchodilator	Asthma
86	Duragesic Patch, Lonsys	Fentanyl	Analgesic (Opioid)	Pain

#	BRAND	GENERIC	CLASS	INDICATION
87	Dyazide, Maxzide	HCTZ + Triamterene	Diuretic (Potassium-sparing and Thiazide)	Hypertension, Edema
88	Dynacin, Minocin, Solodyn	Minocycline	Antibiotic (Tetracycline)	Infection
89	Ecotrin	Aspirin	Antiplatelet, NSAID, Salicylate	Pain, Fever, Stroke, Acute Coronary Syndrome
90	Effexor	Venlafaxine	Antidepressant, SNRI	Depression, Anxiety
91	Elavil	Amitriptyline	Antidepressant (Tricyclic)	Depression
92	Eliquis	Apixaban	Anticoagulant	Stroke, Deep Vein Thrombosis, Pulmonary Embolism
93	Emtriva	Emtricitabine	HIV, NRTI	HIV Infection
94	Errin, Heather, Camila	Norethindrone	Contraceptive	Birth Control
95	Erythrocin	Erythromycin	Antibiotic (Macrolide)	Infection
96	Estrace	Estradiol oral	Estrogen Derivatives	Osteoporosis, Breast Cancer, Prostate Cancer
97	Farxiga	Dapagliflozin	Sodium-glucose cotransporter 2 inhibitor	Diabetes
98	Feosol, Fer-In-Sol	Ferrous Sulfate	Iron Product	Anemia
99	Flagyl	Metronidazole	Antifungal, Bacterial vaginosis, Intestinal infections	Infection
100	Flexeril	Cyclobenzaprine	Skeletal Muscle Relaxant	Muscle Relaxer
101	Flomax	Tamsulosin	Alpha Blocker	Benign Prostate Hyperplasia (BPH)
102	Flonase, Veramyst, Flovent HFA, Arnuity Ellipta, Flovent Diskus	Fluticasone	Intranasal Adrenal Glucocorticosteroid	Asthma, Allergic Rhinitis, Nasal Polyps
103	Focalin	Dexmethylphenidate Hydrochloride	CNS Stimulant	Attention-deficit hyperactivity disorder (ADHD), Narcolepsy

#	BRAND	GENERIC	CLASS	INDICATION
104	Folate, Folvite	Folic Acid	Vitamins, Water-Soluble	Nutritional Supplementation
105	Fosamax	Alendronate	Bisphosphonate	Osteoporosis
106	Geodon	Ziprasidone	Antipsychotic	Schizophrenia, Bipolar, Psychosis
107	Glucophage	Metformin	Biguanide	Diabetes
108	Glucotrol	Glipizide	Antidiabetic, Sulfonylureas	Diabetes
109	Golytely, Miralax	Polyethylene Glycol 3350	Laxative	Constipation, Bowel Preparation
110	Halcion	Triazolam	Sedative, Hypnotic	Insomnia
111	Haldol	Haloperidol	Antipsychotic	Schizophrenia, Psychosis
112	Humalog	Insulin Lispro	Antidiabetic, Insulin, Rapid Acting	Diabetes
113	Humira	Adalimumab	DMARD, Antipsoriatic	Rheumatoid Arthritis, Psoriatic Arthritis, Crohn Disease, Ulcerative Colitis
114	Humulin R, Novolin R	Insulin Human	Antidiabetic, Insulin, Short Acting	Diabetes
115	Hygroton, Thalitone	Chlorthalidone	Diuretic (Thiazide)	Edema, Hypertension, Heart Failure
116	Hytrin	Terazosin	Alpha Blocker	Benign Prostate Hyperplasia (BPH), Hypertension
117	Hyzaar	HCTZ + Losartan	Diuretic + Angiotensin II Receptor Blocker	Hypertension, Edema
118	Imdur	Isosorbide Mononitrate	Nitrate	Angina
119	Imitrex	Sumatriptan	Antimigraine, Serotonin Receptor Agonist	Migraine Headaches
120	Impoyz, Temovate	Clobetasol	Corticosteroid	Psoriasis
121	Inderal	Propranolol	Beta Blocker	Hypertension
122	Indocin, Tivorbex	Indomethacin	Nonsteroidal anti-inflammatory drugs (NSAID)	Pain, Inflammation, Acute Gouty Arthritis
123	Intuniv	Guanfacine	α2-Adrenergic Agonist	Hypertension

#	BRAND	GENERIC	CLASS	INDICATION
124	Invokana	Canagliflozin	Sodium-glucose cotransporter 2 inhibitor	Diabetes
125	Janumet XR	Metformin + Sitagliptin	Antidiabetic, Biguanides + Dipeptyl Peptidase-IV Inhibitor	Diabetes
126	Januvia	Sitagliptin	Antidiabetic, DPP4 Inhibitor	Diabetes
127	Jardiance	Empagliflozin	Antidiabetic, SGLT2 Inhibitor	Diabetes
128	Keflex	Cephalexin	Antibiotic	Infection
129	Kenalog, Trianex, Triacet, Nasacort AQ	Triamcinolone Topical	Corticosteroid	Inflammation
130	Keppra	Levetiracetam	Anticonvulsant	Seizure
131	Klonopin	Clonazepam	Benzodiazepines	Anxiety
132	Klor-Con	Potassium Chloride	Electrolyte Supplements	Hypokalemia
133	Lamictal	Lamotrigine	Anticonvulsant	Seizure, Bipolar disorder
134	Lanoxin	Digoxin	Antiarrhythmic	Heart Failure, Arrhythmia, Atrial fibrillation
135	Lantus	Insulin Glargine	Antidiabetic, Insulin, Long Acting	Diabetes
136	Lasix	Furosemide	Diuretic (Loop)	Edema, Hypertension, Hyperkalemia
137	Latuda	Lurasidone	Antipsychotic	Schizophrenia, Bipolar, Psychosis
138	Levaquin	Levofloxacin	Antibiotic (Fluoroquinolone)	Infection
139	Levemir	Insulin Detemir	Antidiabetic, Insulin, Long Acting	Diabetes
140	Lexapro	Escitalopram	Antidepressant, SSRI	Depression
141	Lidoderm	Lidocaine Patch	Local Anesthetic	Pain
142	Linzess	Linaclotide	Gastrointestinal, IBS Agent	Irritable Bowel Syndrome, Chronic Idiopathic Constipation
143	Lioresal	Baclofen	Skeletal Muscle Relaxant	Muscle Relaxer

#	BRAND	GENERIC	CLASS	INDICATION
144	Lipitor	Atorvastatin	Antihyperlipidemic, HMG-CoA Reductase Inhibitor	Cholesterol
145	Lithobid, Eskalith	Lithium	Antimanic	Bipolar Disorder
146	Lopid	Gemfibrozil	Antihyperlipidemic, Fibric Acid Derivative	Cholesterol, Triglyceride
147	Lotensin	Benazepril	Angiotensin-converting enzyme (ACE) Inhibitor	Hypertension
148	Lotrel	Amlodipine + Benazepril	Calcium Channel Blocker + Angiotensin-converting enzyme (ACE) Inhibitor	Hypertension
149	Lotrisone	Betamethasone Dipropionate + Clotrimazole	Corticosteroid, Antifungal	Tinea Cruris, Tinea Corporis, Tinea Pedis
150	Lovaza	Omega-3 Fatty Acid Ethyl Esters	Antihyperlipidemic	High Triglyceride
151	Lovenox	Enoxaparin	Anticoagulant	Stroke, Deep Vein Thrombosis, Angina, Acute Coronary Syndromes
152	Lumigan	Bimatoprost	Antiglaucoma	Glaucoma
153	Lunesta	Eszopiclone	Sedative	Insomnia
154	Lyrica	Pregabalin	Anticonvulsant, Analgesic	Seizure, Neuropathic Pain
155	Macrobid, Macrodantin	Nitrofurantoin	Antibiotic	Infection
156	Mag-Ox 400	Magnesium Oxide	Antacid, Electrolyte	Antacid, Magnesium Supplementation
157	Maxalt	Rizatriptan	Antimigraine, Serotonin Receptor Agonist	Migraine Headaches
158	Medrol	Methylprednisolone	Corticosteroid, Anti-inflammatory	Inflammation, Allergic Condition
159	Mevacor, Altoprev	Lovastatin	Antihyperlipidemic, HMG-CoA Reductase Inhibitor	Cholesterol
160	Micardis	Telmisartan	Angiotensin II Receptor Blocker	Hypertension

#	BRAND	GENERIC	CLASS	INDICATION
161	Micronase, Diabeta	Glyburide	Antidiabetic, Sulfonylureas	Diabetes
162	Microzide	Hydrochlorothiazide (HCTZ)	Diuretic (Thiazide)	Edema, Hypertension
163	Minipress, Prazo, Prazin	Prazosin	Alpha Blocker	Hypertension
164	Mirapex	Pramipexole	Antiparkinson Agent, Dopamine Agonist	Parkinson Disease
165	Mobic	Meloxicam	Nonsteroidal anti-inflammatory drugs (NSAID)	Osteoarthritis
166	Motrin, Advil	Ibuprofen	Nonsteroidal anti-inflammatory drugs (NSAID)	Pain, Fever, Inflammation
167	MS Contin, Avinza, Kadian	Morphine Sulfate	Analgesic (Opioid)	Pain
168	Mucinex	Guaifenesin	Expectorant	Cough
169	Mycostatin, Nyamyc, Nystop	Nystatin	Antifungal	Infection
170	Myrbetriq	Mirabegron	Beta 3 Agonist	Overactive Bladder
171	Mysoline	Primidone	Anticonvulsant	Seizure
172	Namenda	Memantine	NMDA Antagonist	Alzheimer Disease, Dementia
173	Naphcon-A, Opcon-A, Visine-A	Naphazoline + Pheniramine	Antihistamine + Decongestant	Allergic Conjunctivitis
174	Nasonex	Mometasone Nasal	Corticosteroid	Allergic Rhinitis
175	Necon 777	Ethinyl Estradiol + Norethindrone	Contraceptive	Birth Control
176	Neoral, Sandimmune, Gengraf	Cyclosporine	Immunosuppressant, DMARD, Calcineurin Inhibitor	Solid Organ Transplantation, Rheumatoid Arthritis, Psoriasis
177	Neosporin	Bacitracin + Neomycin + Polymyxin B	Antibiotic	Infection
178	Neurontin	Gabapentin	Anticonvulsant	Seizure, Neuralgia
179	Nexium	Esomeprazole	Proton Pump Inhibitor	Gastroesophageal Reflux Disease (GERD), Ulcers, Erosive Esophagitis
180	Niaspan, Slo-Niacin	Niacin	Antihyperlipidemic	Cholesterol

#	BRAND	GENERIC	CLASS	INDICATION
181	Nitrostat, Minitran	Nitroglycerin	Nitrate, Vasodilator	Angina
182	Nizoral	Ketoconazole Topical	Antifungal	Infection
183	Norco, Vicodin, Lorcet	Acetaminophen + Hydrocodone	Analgesic (Narcotic)	Pain
184	Normodyne	Labetalol	Beta Blocker	Hypertension
185	Norvasc	Amlodipine	Calcium Channel Blocker	Hypertension
186	Novolog	Insulin Aspart	Antidiabetic, Insulin, Rapid Acting	Diabetes
187	NuvaRing	Ethinyl Estradiol + Etonogestrel	Contraceptive	Birth Control
188	Ocean, Ayr Saline	Sodium Chloride	Decongestant, Intranasal	Congestion, Nasal Dryness
189	Ocuflox	Ofloxacin	Antibiotic (Quinolone)	Infection, Bacterial Conjunctivitis, Corneal Ulcer
190	Omnicef	Cefdinir	Antibiotic	Infection
191	Orapred, Prelone, Pediapred	Prednisolone Oral	Glucocorticosteroid	Rheumatoid Arthritis, Multiple Sclerosis
192	Os-Cal Ultra, Caltrate 600 + D3	Calcium + Cholecalciferol	Vitamins, Fat-Soluble	Calcium Supplementation
193	OxyContin	Oxycodone	Analgesic (Opioid)	Pain
194	Pamelor	Nortriptyline	Antidepressant (Tricyclic)	Depression
195	Patanol, Pataday	Olopatadine	Antihistamine	Allergic Conjunctivitis
196	Paxil	Paroxetine	Antidepressant, SSRI	Depression, Obsessive-Compulsive Disorder, Anxiety
197	Pen Vee K, Penicillin V	Penicillin VK	Antibiotic (Penicillin)	Infection
198	Pepcid	Famotidine	Histamine H2 Antagonist	Heartburn
199	Peridex, PerioGard, PerioChip	Chlorhexidine	Antibiotic	Antibacterial Cleansing Agent
200	Phenergan	Promethazine	Antihistamine, Antiemetic	Nausea and Vomiting, Motion Sickness, Sedation, Allergy

#	BRAND	GENERIC	CLASS	INDICATION
201	Phrenilin Forte, Phrenilin, Bupap, Orbivan CF	Acetaminophen + Butalbital	Analgesic + Barbiturate Combo	Pain
202	Plaquenil	Hydroxychloroquine	Aminoquinoline	Lupus, Rheumatoid Arthritis, Malaria
203	Plavix	Clopidogrel	Antiplatelet	Stroke, Acute Coronary Syndrome
204	Pravachol	Pravastatin	Antihyperlipidemic, HMG-CoA Reductase Inhibitor	Cholesterol
205	Premarin	Estrogens, Conjugated	Estrogen Derivatives	Menopause, Female Hypogonadism, Osteoporosis, Prostate Cancer, Abnormal Uterine Bleeding
206	Prempro	Conjugated Estrogens + Medroxyprogesterone	Hormone Replacement	Menopause
207	Prevacid	Lansoprazole	Proton Pump Inhibitor	Gastroesophageal Reflux Disease (GERD), Ulcers, Erosive Esophagitis
208	PreviDent	Sodium Fluoride	Oral Rinse	Dental Caries Prevention
209	Prilosec	Omeprazole	Proton Pump Inhibitor	Gastroesophageal Reflux Disease (GERD), Ulcers
210	Prinivil, Zestril	Lisinopril	Angiotensin-converting enzyme (ACE) Inhibitor	Hypertension
211	Pristiq	Desvenlafaxine	Serotonin/Norepinephrine Reuptake Inhibitor	Depression
212	Proair HFA, Proventil HFA, Ventolin HFA	Albuterol	Bronchodilator	Asthma
213	Procardia, Adalat	Nifedipine	Calcium Channel Blocker	Hypertension
214	Prometrium	Progesterone	Progestin Hormone	Prevention of Endometrial Hyperplasia, Secondary Amenorrhea

#	BRAND	GENERIC	CLASS	INDICATION
215	Proscar, Propecia	Finasteride	5-Alpha-Reductase Inhibitor	Benign Prostate Hyperplasia (BPH)
216	Protonix	Pantoprazole	Proton Pump Inhibitor	Gastroesophageal Reflux Disease (GERD)
217	Provera, Depo-Provera	Medroxyprogesterone	Progestin hormone	Abnormal Uterine Bleeding, Contraception
218	Prozac	Fluoxetine	Antidepressant, SSRI	Depression, Anxiety
219	Pulmicort Flexhaler	Budesonide	Corticosteroid	Asthma
220	Qvar	Beclomethasone Dipropionate	Corticosteroid	Asthma
221	Ranexa	Ranolazine	Antianginal, Non-nitrates	Angina
222	Reglan	Metoclopramide	Antiemetic, Prokinetic	Nausea and Vomiting, Diabetic Gastroparesis, GERD
223	Remeron	Mirtazapine	Antidepressant, Serotonin and α_2-adrenergic Antagonist	Depression
224	Requip	Ropinirole	Antiparkinson Agent, Dopamine Agonist	Parkinson Disease, Restless Leg Syndrome
225	Restoril	Temazepam	Sedative, Hypnotic	Insomnia
226	Retin A	Tretinoin	Acne Agent	Acne
227	Risperdal	Risperidone	Antipsychotic, Antimanic	Schizophrenia, Bipolar, Psychosis
228	Ritalin, Concerta	Methylphenidate	CNS Stimulant	Attention-deficit hyperactivity disorder (ADHD), Narcolepsy
229	Robaxin	Methocarbamol	Skeletal Muscle Relaxant	Muscle Relaxer
230	Rocaltrol	Calcitriol	Vitamin D Analogs	Calcium Deficiency with Hypoparathyroidism
231	Senna, Senokot	Sennosides	Laxative	Constipation
232	Seroquel	Quetiapine	Antipsychotic, Antimanic	Schizophrenia, Bipolar, Psychosis, Depression
233	Sinemet, Sinemet CR	Carbidopa + Levodopa	Antiparkinson Agent	Parkinson Disease
234	Sinequan, Silenor	Doxepin	Antidepressant (Tricyclic)	Depression, Anxiety, Insomnia
235	Singulair	Montelukast	Leukotriene Inhibitor	Asthma, Bronchospasm, Allergic Rhinitis

#	BRAND	GENERIC	CLASS	INDICATION
236	Soltamox	Tamoxifen	Antineoplastic	Breast Cancer
237	Soma	Carisoprodol	Skeletal Muscle Relaxant	Muscle Relaxer
238	Spiriva Handihaler	Tiotropium	Bronchodilator	Asthma, Chronic Obstructive Pulmonary Disease (COPD)
239	Strattera	Atomoxetine	CNS Stimulant	Attention-deficit hyperactivity disorder (ADHD), Narcolepsy
240	Suboxone, Bunavail, Zubsolv	Buprenorphine + Naloxone	Opioid partial agonist and antagonist combination	Opioid Dependence
241	Symbicort	Budesonide + Formoterol	Respiratory Inhalant Combo	Asthma, Chronic Obstructive Pulmonary Disease (COPD)
242	Synthroid	Levothyroxine	Thyroid	Hypothyroidism
243	Tambacor	Flecainide	Antiarrhythmic	Arrhythmias
244	Tamiflu	Oseltamivir	Antiviral	Influenza A and B
245	Tapazole	Methimazole	Thyroid	Hyperthyroidism, Graves Disease
246	Tegretol	Carbamazepine	Anticonvulsant	Seizure, Bipolar disorder
247	Tenoretic	Atenolol + Chlorthalidone	Beta Blocker + Diuretic	Hypertension, Edema
248	Tenormin	Atenolol	Beta Blocker	Hypertension
249	Tessalon Perles	Benzonatate	Antitussive	Cough
250	Timoptic	Timolol	Antiglaucoma, Beta Blocker	Ocular Hypertension
251	Topamax	Topiramate	Anticonvulsant	Seizure, Migraine Headache
252	Toprol XL, Lopressor	Metoprolol	Beta Blocker	Hypertension
253	Toradol	Ketorolac	Nonsteroidal anti-inflammatory drugs (NSAID)	Pain
254	Tradjenta	Linagliptin	Dipeptidyl Peptidase 4 Inhibitor	Diabetes
255	Travatan Z	Travoprost	Antiglaucoma	Glaucoma
256	Tresiba	Insulin Degludec	Antidiabetic, Insulin, Long Acting	Diabetes

#	BRAND	GENERIC	CLASS	INDICATION
257	Trexall	Methotrexate	Immunosuppressant, Antineoplstic, DMARD	Rheumatoid Arthritis, Psoriasis, Cancer, Neoplasms, Leukemia
258	Tricor, Trilipix, Antara, Fenoglide, Lipofen, Lofibra, Trilipix	Fenofibrate	Antihyperlipidemic, Fibric Acid Derivative	Cholesterol
259	Trileptal	Oxcarbazepine	Anticonvulsant	Seizure
260	Trinessa-28, Ortho Tri-Cyclen, Ortho Tri-Cyclen Lo	Ethinyl Estradiol + Norgestimate	Contraceptive	Birth Control
261	Trulicity	Dulaglutide	Glucagon-Like Peptide-1 Receptor Agonist	Diabetes
262	Trusopt	Dorzolamide	Antiglaucoma	Glaucoma, Ocular Hypertension
263	Tums, Oysco	Calcium	Antacid	Calcium Supplementation, Heart burn
264	Twirla	Ethinyl Estradiol + Levonorgestrel	Contraceptive	Birth Control
265	Tylenol	Acetaminophen	Analgesic	Pain
266	Ultram	Tramadol	Analgesic (Opioid)	Pain
267	Uroxatral	Alfuzosin	Alpha Blocker	Benign Prostate Hyperplasia (BPH), Hypertension
268	Valium	Diazepam	Benzodiazepines, Sedative	Anxiety, Sleep, Muscle Relaxer
269	Valtrex	Valacyclovir	Antiviral	Infection
270	Vasotec	Enalapril	Angiotensin-converting enzyme (ACE) Inhibitor	Hypertension
271	Vesicare	Solifenacin	Anticholinergic, Genitourinary	Overactive Bladder
272	Viagra, Revatio	Sildenafil	Phosphodiesterase-5 (PDE-5) Enzyme Inhibitor	Erectile Dysfunction, Pulmonary Arterial Hypertension
273	Vibramycin	Doxycycline	Antibiotic (Tetracycline)	Infection

#	BRAND	GENERIC	CLASS	INDICATION
274	Victoza, Saxenda	Liraglutide	Glucagon-Like Peptide-1 Receptor Agonist	Diabetes
275	Viibryd	Vilazodone	Antidepressant, Mixed serotonergic effects	Depression
276	Vitamin B12	Cyanocobalamin	Vitamins, Water-Soluble	Nutritional Supplementation
277	Vitamin D	Ergocalciferol	Vitamins, Fat-Soluble	Nutritional Supplementation
278	Voltaren, Cambia, Zipsor, Zorvolex	Diclofenac Sodium	Nonsteroidal anti-inflammatory drugs (NSAID)	Pain, Osteoarthritis, Rheumatoid Arthritis
279	Vytorin	Ezetimibe + Simvastatin	Antihyperlipidemic	Cholesterol
280	Vyvanse	Lisdexamfetamine	CNS stimulant	Attention-deficit hyperactivity disorder (ADHD), Narcolepsy
281	Wellbutrin, Zyban	Bupropion	Antidepressant, Smoking Cessation Aids	Depression, Smoking Cessation
282	Xalatan	Latanoprost	Prostaglandin	Glaucoma
283	Xanax	Alprazolam	Benzodiazepines, Antianxiety, Anxiolytic	Anxiety
284	Xarelto	Rivaroxaban	Anticoagulant, Factor Xa Inhibitor	Stroke, Deep Vein Thrombosis, Pulmonary Embolism
285	Xyzal	Levocetirizine	Antihistamine	Allergic Rhinitis, Urticaria
286	Yaz	Drospirenone + Ethinyl estradiol	Contraceptive	Birth Control
287	Zanaflex	Tizanidine	Alpha 2 Adrenergic Agonist	Muscle Relaxer
288	Zantac	Ranitidine	Histamine H2 Antagonist	Gastroesophageal Reflux Disease (GERD)
289	Zebeta	Bisoprolol	Beta Blocker	Hypertension
290	Zestoretic	Hydrochlorothiazide (HCTZ) + Lisinopril	Diuretic + Angiotensin-converting enzyme (ACE) Inhibitor	Hypertension, Edema
291	Zetia	Ezetimibe	Antihyperlipidemic	Cholesterol

#	BRAND	GENERIC	CLASS	INDICATION
292	Zocor	Simvastatin	Antihyperlipidemic, HMG-CoA Reductase Inhibitor	Cholesterol
293	Zofran	Ondansetron	Antiemetic	Nausea and Vomiting
294	Zohydro ER, Hysingla ER, Vantrela ER	Hydrocodone Bitartrate	Analgesic (Opioid)	Pain
295	Zoloft	Sertraline	Antidepressant, SSRI	Depression, Anxiety, Obsessive-Compulsive Disorder, PTSD
296	Zovirax	Acyclovir	Antiviral	Infection
297	Z-Pak, Zithromax	Azithromycin	Antibiotic (Macrolide)	Infection
298	Zyloprim	Allopurinol	Xanthine Oxidase Inhibitor	Gout
299	Zyprexa	Olanzapine	Antipsychotic, Antimanic	Schizophrenia, Bipolar, Psychosis
300	Zyrtec	Cetirizine	Antihistamine	Allergy, Hay Fever, Urticaria

19.

❧

BOXED WARNING MEDS IN ALPHABETICAL ORDER BY BRAND

Boxed warning, also known as black box warning, appears on medications that has serious or life-threatening risks.

#	BRAND	GENERIC
1	Abilify	Aripiprazole
2	Accupril	Quinapril
3	Actos	Pioglitazone
4	Adderall	Amphetamine + Dextroamphetamine
5	Advair	Fluticasone + Salmeterol
6	Aldactone	Spironolactone
7	Altace	Ramipril
8	Ambien	Zolpidem
9	Anaprox	Naproxen
10	Androgel	Testosterone Gel
11	Armour Thyroid	Thyroid
12	Ativan	Lorazepam
13	Avapro	Irbesartan
14	Benicar	Olmesartan

#	BRAND	GENERIC
15	Benicar HCT	Olmesartan + HCTZ
16	Betapace, Sorine	Sotalol
17	Brilinta	Ticagrelor
18	Bumex, Burinex	Bumetanide
19	Byetta, Bydureon	Exenatide
20	Celebrex	Celecoxib
21	Celexa	Citalopram
22	CellCept, Myfortic	Mycophenolate
23	Cipro	Ciprofloxacin
24	Cleocin	Clindamycin
25	Cordarone	Amiodarone
26	Coumadin	Warfarin
27	Cozaar	Losartan
28	Cymbalta	Duloxetine
29	Cytomel	Liothyronine
30	Depakote, Depakote ER	Divalproex Sodium
31	Depo Provera	Medroxyprogesterone
32	Desyrel	Trazodone
33	Dilantin	Phenytoin
34	Dilaudid	Hydromorphone
35	Diovan	Valsartan
36	Diovan HCT	Valsartan + HCTZ
37	Duragesic Patch, Lonsys	Fentanyl
38	Dyazide, Maxzide	Triamterene + HCTZ
39	Effexor	Venlafaxine
40	Elavil	Amitriptyline
41	Eliquis	Apixaban
42	Emtriva	Emtricitabine
43	Estrace	Estradiol topical
44	Flagyl	Metronidazole
45	Focalin	Dexmethylphenidate Hydrochloride
46	Geodon	Ziprasidone

#	BRAND	GENERIC
47	Glucophage	Metformin
48	Halcion	Triazolam
49	Haldol	Haloperidol
50	Humira	Adalimumab
51	Hyzaar	Losartan + HCTZ
52	Inderal	Propranolol
53	Indocin, Tivorbex	Indomethacin
54	Janumet XR	Metformin + Sitagliptin
55	Klonopin	Clonazepam
56	Lamictal	Lamotrigine
57	Lasix	Furosemide
58	Latuda	Lurasidone
59	Levaquin	Levofloxacin
60	Lexapro	Escitalopram
61	Linzess	Linaclotide
62	Lioresal	Baclofen
63	Lithobid, Eskalith	Lithium
64	Lopressor	Metoprolol Tartrate
65	Lotensin	Benazepril
66	Lotrel	Amlodipine + Benazepril
67	Lovenox	Enoxaparin
68	Lunesta	Eszopiclone
69	Micardis	Telmisartan
70	Mobic	Meloxicam
71	Motrin, Advil	Ibuprofen
72	MS Contin, Avinza, Kadian	Morphine
73	Necon 777	Ethinyl Estradiol + Norethindrone
74	Neoral, Sandimmune, Gengraf	Cyclosporine
75	Nizoral	Ketoconazole
76	Norco	Hydrocodone + Acetaminophen
77	NuvaRing	Ethinyl Estradiol + Etonogestrel Vaginal Ring
78	OxyContin	Oxycodone

#	BRAND	GENERIC
79	Pamelor	Nortiptyline
80	Paxil	Paroxetine
81	Percocet, Endocet, Roxicet	Oxycodone + Acetaminophen
82	Phenergan	Promethazine
83	Plavix	Clopidogrel
84	Premarin	Conjugated Estrogens
85	Prinivil, Zestril	Lisinopril
86	Prinzide, Zestoretic	Lisinopril + HCTZ
87	Pristiq	Desvenlafaxine
88	Prometrium	Progesterone
89	Prozac	Fluoxetine
90	Reglan	Metoclopramide
91	Remeron	Mirtazapine
92	Restoril	Temazepam
93	Ritalin, Concerta	Methylphenidate
94	Seroquel	Quetiapine
95	Sinequan, Silenor	Doxepin
96	Singulair	Montelukast
97	Soltamox	Tamoxifen
98	Strattera	Atomoxetine
99	Symbicort	Budesonide + Formoterol
100	Synthroid, Levoxyl, Levothroid	Levothyroxine
101	Tambacor	Flecainide
102	Tegretol	Carbamazepine
103	Tenormin	Atenolol
104	Toprol XL	Metoprolol Succinate
105	Toradol	Ketorolac
106	Trexall	Methotrexate
107	Trinessa-28, Ortho Tri-Cyclen, Ortho Tri-Cyclen Lo	Ethinyl Estradiol + Norgestimate
108	Trulicity	Dulaglutide
109	Ultram	Tramadol
110	Valium	Diazepam

#	BRAND	GENERIC
111	Vasotec	Enalapril
112	Victoza	Liraglutide
113	Viibryd	Vilazodone
114	Vyvanse	Lisdexamfetamine
115	Wellbutrin, Zyban	Bupropion
116	Xanax	Alprazolam
117	Xarelto	Rivaroxaban
118	Yaz	Ethinyl Estradiol + Drospirenone
119	Zoloft	Sertraline
120	Zyprexa	Olanzapine

PART 4

EXTRA MEDICATIONS

20.

ADDITIONAL 100 MEDS

Acne

CLASS: Acne Agent		
#	GENERIC	BRAND
1	Adapalene	Differin
2	Benzoyl Peroxide + Clindamycin	Benzaclin
3	Isotretinoin	Zenatane

Diabetes

CLASS: Antidiabetic			
#	GENERIC	BRAND	SUBCLASS
1	Insulin Glulisine	Apidra	Insulin, Rapid Acting
2	Insulin NPH	Humulin N, Novolin N	Insulin, Intermediate Acting
3	Insulin NPH (70%), Regular (30%)	Humulin 70/30, Novolin 70/30	Insulin mix
4	Insulin Aspart Protamine (70%), Aspart (30%)	NovoLog Mix 70/30	Insulin mix
5	Saxagliptin	Onglyza	DPP4 Inhibitor
6	Nateglinide	Starlix	Meglitinides
7	Repaglinide	Prandin	Meglitinides
8	Rosiglitazone	Avandia	Thiazolidinediones

Eye Drop and Ear Drop

#	GENERIC	BRAND	CLASS
1	Gatifloxacin	Zymar, Zymaxid	Antibiotic
2	Loteprednol	Alrex, Lotemax	Corticosteroid
3	Moxifloxacin	Vigamox,	Antibiotic
4	Tobramycin	Tobrex	Antibiotic
5	Ciprofloxacin + Dexamethasone Otic (Ear Drop)	Ciprodex	Antibiotic + Corticosteroid

HIV Infection

CLASS: Antiretroviral		
#	GENERIC	BRAND
1	Maraviroc	Selzentry
2	Atazanavir	Reyataz
3	Efavirenz	Sustiva
4	Emtricitabine + Tenofovir	Truvada
5	Entecavir	Baraclude
6	Raltegravir	Isentress
7	Abacavir + Lamivudine	Epzicom

Hypertension

CLASS: Antihypertensive		
#	GENERIC	BRAND	SUBCLASS
1	Candesartan	Atacand	ARB
2	Candesartan + HCTZ	Atacand-HCT	ARB + Diuretic
3	Elmisartan + HCTZ	Micardis-HCT	ARB + Diuretic
4	Irbesartan + HCTZ	Avalide	ARB + Diuretic
5	Captopril	Capoten	ACE Inhibitor
6	Fosinopril	Monopril	ACE Inhibitor
7	Perindopril	Aceon	ACE Inhibitor
8	Felodipine	Plendil	CCB

9	Amlodipine + Olmesartan	Azor	CCB + ARB
10	Amlodipine + Valsartan	Exforge	CCB + ARB
11	Aliskiren	Tekturna	Renin Inhibitor
12	Sacubitril + Valsartan	Entresto	Neprilysin Inhibitor + ARB

Infection

CLASS: Antibiotic		
#	GENERIC	BRAND
1	Cefaclor	Ceclor
2	Cefazolin	Ancef
3	Cefprozil	Cefzil
4	Cefuroxime	Ceftin
5	Clarithromycin	Biaxin
6	Vancomycin	Vancocin

Inflammation, Allergy

CLASS: Corticosteroid		
#	GENERIC	BRAND
1	Dexamethasone	Decadron
2	Fluocinonide Topical	Lidex
3	Methylprednisolone	Medrol

Migraine Headache

CLASS: Antimigraine		
#	GENERIC	BRAND
1	Butalbital + Caffeine + Acetaminophen	Fioricet
2	Butalbital + Caffeine + Aspirin	Fiorinal
3	Eletriptan	Relpax
4	Zolmitriptan	Zomig

Seizure

CLASS: Anticonvulsant		
#	GENERIC	BRAND
1	Clobazam	Onfi
2	Lacosamide	Vimpat
3	Phenobarbital	Luminal

Motion Sickness, Nausea and Vomiting

CLASS: Antiemetic		
#	GENERIC	BRAND
1	Scopolamine	Transdermscop
2	Prochlorperazine	Compazine

Pain, Osteoarthritis, Rheumatoid Arthritis

CLASS: Nonsteroidal anti-inflammatory drugs (NSAID)		
#	GENERIC	BRAND
1	Etodolac	Lodine
2	Nabumetone	Relafen
3	Piroxicam	Feldene

Pain

CLASS: Analgesic		
#	GENERIC	BRAND
1	Phenazopyridine	Pyridium
2	Hydrocodone + Ibuprofen	Vicoprofen
3	Meperidine	Demerol
4	Acetaminophen + Codeine	Tylenol with Codeine
5	Acetaminophen + Oxycodone	Percocet
6	Acetaminophen + Tramadol	Ultracet
7	Methadone	Dolophine

Osteoporosis Medications

#	GENERIC	BRAND	CLASS
1	Ibandronate	Boniva	Bisphosphonate
2	Risedronate	Actonel, Atelvia	Bisphosphonate
3	Raloxifene	Evista	Selective Estrogen Receptor Modulator (SERM)

Insomnia

CLASS: Sedative	
#	GENERIC	BRAND
---	---------	-------
1	Zaleplon	Sonata
2	Ramelteon	Rozerem

Vaccine

#	GENERIC	BRAND
1	Hepatitis A Vaccine	Havrix, Vaqta
2	Hepatitis B Vaccine	Engerix-B, Recombivax HB
3	Herpes Zoster Vaccine	Zostavax, Shingrix
4	Human Papillomavirus Vaccine	Gardasil 9
5	Influenza Vaccine	Afluria, Fluad, Fluzone, Fluarix
6	Measles, Mumps, Rubella Vaccine	MMR-II
7	Meningococcal Vaccine	Menactra, Menveo Trumenba, Bexero
8	Pneumococcal Vaccine	Prevnar 13, Pneumovax 23
9	Polio Vaccine	Ipol
10	Rotavirus Vaccine	Rotarix, RotaTeq
11	Tdap (Tetanus, Diphtheria, Pertussis)	Daptacel, Adacel, Boostrix, Infanrix

MISCELLANEOUS

#	GENERIC	BRAND	CLASS	INDICATION
1	Azathioprine	Azamun, Imuran	Immunosuppressant	Kidney Transplant, Rheumatoid Arthritis
2	Cinacalcet	Sensipar	Calcimimetics	Hyperparathyroidism, Parathyroid Carcinoma
3	Clorazepate	Tranxene-T	Sedative, Anxiety, Anticonvulsant	Anxiety, Seizure
4	Colesevelam	Welchol	Bile Acid Sequestrant	Cholesterol, Diabetes
5	Dabigatran	Pradaxa	Anticoagulant	Stroke, Deep Vein Thrombosis and Pulmonary Embolus
6	Diphenoxylate and Atropine	Lomotil	Antidiarrhea	Diarrhea
7	Febuxostat	Uloric	Xanthine Oxidase Inhibitor	Gout
8	Fexofenadine + Pseudoephedrine	Allegra-D	Antihistamine + Decongestant	Allergic Rhinitis, Nasal Congestion
9	Fluvoxamine	Luvox	Antidepressant, SSRI	Depression, Anxiety
10	Imiquimod	Zyclara, Aldara	Immune Response Modifier	External Genital Warts
11	Levalbuterol	Xopenex HFA	Bronchodilator	Asthma
12	Lubiprostone	Amitiza	Chloride Channel Activator	Constipation
13	Rifaximin	Xifaxan	Antibiotic, Antidiarrheal	Traveler's Diarrhea, Hepatic Encephalopathy, Irritable Bowel Syndrome
14	Sevelamer carbonate	Renvela	Phosphate Binder	High Phosphate Level in dialysis patient
15	Tacrolimus	Prograf	Immunosuppressants, Calcineurin Inhibitor	Transplant (Heart, Liver, Kidney)
16	Terbinafine	Lamisil	Antifungal	Nail Fungus
17	Ticagrelor	Brilinta	Antiplatelet	Acute Coronary Syndrome

18	Tropium	Sanctura	Anticholinergic	Overactive Bladder
19	Vardenafil	Levitra	Phosphodiesterase Inhibitor	Erectile Dysfunction
20	Varenicline	Chantix	Smoking Cessation Aids	Smoking Cessation

PART 5

PRACTICE

21.

⸻ ❧ ⸻

PRACTICE MAKES
PROGRESS

They say repetition is the mother of skills. Doing more practice is probably the best way to ensure the retention of those medication names in your memory. This part of the book allows you to do just that by recalling what you have learned so far.

There are four tables in total. The first three tables let you practice on the top 300 medications while the fourth one contains the extra one hundred medications in alphabetical order by generic names.

By Rank (Top 300)

Fill out the brand names of the following generic medications

Rank	GENERIC	BRAND
1	Lisinopril	
2	Atorvastatin	
3	Levothyroxine	
4	Metformin	
5	Amlodipine	
6	Metoprolol	
7	Omeprazole	
8	Simvastatin	
9	Losartan	
10	Albuterol	
11	Gabapentin	
12	Hydrochlorothiazide	
13	Acetaminophen + Hydrocodone	
14	Sertraline	
15	Fluticasone	
16	Montelukast	
17	Furosemide	
18	Amoxicillin	
19	Pantoprazole	
20	Escitalopram	
21	Alprazolam	
22	Prednisone	
23	Bupropion	
24	Pravastatin	
25	Acetaminophen	
26	Citalopram	

Rank	GENERIC	BRAND
27	Dextroamphetamine + Amphetamine	
28	Ibuprofen	
29	Carvedilol	
30	Trazodone	
31	Fluoxetine	
32	Tramadol	
33	Insulin Glargine	
34	Clonazepam	
35	Tamsulosin	
36	Atenolol	
37	Potassium	
38	Meloxicam	
39	Rosuvastatin	
40	Clopidogrel	
41	Propranolol	
42	Aspirin	
43	Cyclobenzaprine	
44	Hydrochlorothiazide + Lisinopril	
45	Glipizide	
46	Duloxetine	
47	Methylphenidate	
48	Ranitidine	
49	Venlafaxine	
50	Zolpidem	
51	Warfarin	
52	Oxycodone	
53	Ethinyl Estradiol + Norethindrone	
54	Allopurinol	
55	Ergocalciferol	
56	Insulin Aspart	

Rank	GENERIC	BRAND
57	Azithromycin	
58	Metronidazole	
59	Loratadine	
60	Lorazepam	
61	Estradiol	
62	Ethinyl Estradiol + Norgestimate	
63	Lamotrigine	
64	Glimepiride	
65	Fluticasone + Salmeterol	
66	Cetirizine	
67	Hydrochlorothiazide + Losartan	
68	Paroxetine	
69	Spironolactone	
70	Fenofibrate	
71	Naproxen	
72	Pregabalin	
73	Insulin Human	
74	Budesonide + Formoterol	
75	Diltiazem	
76	Quetiapine	
77	Topiramate	
78	Bacitracin + Neomycin + Polymyxin B	
79	Clonidine	
80	Buspirone	
81	Latanoprost	
82	Tiotropium	
83	Ondansetron	
84	Lovastatin	
85	Valsartan	
86	Finasteride	

Rank	GENERIC	BRAND
87	Amitriptyline	
88	Esomeprazole	
89	Tizanidine	
90	Alendronate	
91	Lisdexamfetamine	
92	Ferrous Sulfate	
93	Apixaban	
94	Diclofenac	
95	Sitagliptin	
96	Folic Acid	
97	Sumatriptan	
98	Drospirenone + Ethinyl Estradiol	
99	Hydroxyzine	
100	Oxybutynin	
101	Hydrochlorothiazide + Triamterene	
102	Cephalexin	
103	Triamcinolone	
104	Benazepril	
105	Hydralazine	
106	Celecoxib	
107	Ciprofloxacin	
108	Ropinirole	
109	Rivaroxaban	
110	Levetiracetam	
111	Isosorbide Mononitrate	
112	Aripiprazole	
113	Doxycycline	
114	Insulin Detemir	
115	Famotidine	
116	Amoxicillin + Clavulanate	

Rank	GENERIC	BRAND
117	Methotrexate	
118	Hydrocodone Bitartrate	
119	Mirtazapine	
120	Nifedipine	
121	Sulfamethoxazole + Trimethoprim	
122	Enalapril	
123	Docusate	
124	Insulin Lispro	
125	Pioglitazone	
126	Divalproex	
127	Donepezil	
128	Hydroxychloroquine	
129	Prednisolone	
130	Thyroid	
131	Guanfacine	
132	Testosterone	
133	Hydrochlorothiazide + Valsartan	
134	Ramipril	
135	Diazepam	
136	Ethinyl Estradiol + Levonorgestrel	
137	Clindamycin	
138	Gemfibrozil	
139	Metformin + Sitagliptin	
140	Baclofen	
141	Norethindrone	
142	Temazepam	
143	Nitroglycerin	
144	Nebivolol	
145	Verapamil	
146	Timolol	

Rank	GENERIC	BRAND
147	Promethazine	
148	Benzonatate	
149	Memantine	
150	Doxazosin	
151	Ezetimibe	
152	Valacyclovir	
153	Beclomethasone	
154	Hydrocortisone	
155	Morphine	
156	Risperidone	
157	Methylprednisolone	
158	Omega-3-acid Ethyl Esters	
159	Oseltamivir	
160	Amlodipine + Benazepril	
161	Meclizine	
162	Polyethylene Glycol 3350	
163	Liraglutide	
164	Desogestrel + Ethinyl Estradiol	
165	Levofloxacin	
166	Acyclovir	
167	Brimonidine	
168	Digoxin	
169	Adalimumab	
170	Cyanocobalamin	
171	Magnesium	
172	Albuterol + Ipratropium	
173	Chlorthalidone	
174	Glyburide	
175	Levocetirizine	
176	Carbamazepine	

Rank	GENERIC	BRAND
177	Ethinyl Estradiol + Etonogestrel	
178	Methocarbamol	
179	Pramipexole	
180	Lithium	
181	Dicyclomine	
182	Fluconazole	
183	Nortriptyline	
184	Carbidopa + Levodopa	
185	Nitrofurantoin	
186	Mupirocin	
187	Acetaminophen + Butalbital	
188	Lansoprazole	
189	Dexmethylphenidate	
190	Budesonide	
191	Mirabegron	
192	Canagliflozin	
193	Menthol	
194	Terazosin	
195	Progesterone	
196	Amiodarone	
197	Mometasone	
198	Cefdinir	
199	Atomoxetine	
200	Linagliptin	
201	Colchicine	
202	Dexlansoprazole	
203	Naphazoline + Pheniramine	
204	Rizatriptan Benzoate	
205	Hydromorphone	
206	Estrogens, Conjugated	

Rank	GENERIC	BRAND
207	Oxcarbazepine	
208	Lidocaine	
209	Clobetasol Propionate	
210	Phentermine	
211	Labetalol	
212	Travoprost	
213	Guaifenesin + Codeine+ Pseudoephedrine	
214	Eszopiclone	
215	Erythromycin	
216	Ipratropium	
217	Sildenafil	
218	Sucralfate	
219	Ketoconazole	
220	Irbesartan	
221	Phenytoin	
222	Medroxyprogesterone	
223	Olmesartan	
224	Emtricitabine	
225	Sodium	
226	Benztropine	
227	Prazosin	
228	Empagliflozin	
229	Tolterodine	
230	Nystatin	
231	Bimatoprost	
232	Dulaglutide	
233	Dorzolamide + Timolol	
234	Guaifenesin	
235	Desvenlafaxine	
236	Calcium + Cholecalciferol	

Rank	GENERIC	BRAND
237	Minocycline	
238	Primidone	
239	Olanzapine	
240	Doxepin	
241	Diphenhydramine	
242	Penicillin V	
243	Formoterol + Mometasone	
244	Methimazole	
245	Fexofenadine	
246	Mesalamine	
247	Sodium Fluoride	
248	Cyclosporine	
249	Telmisartan	
250	Fentanyl	
251	Tamoxifen	
252	Liothyronine	
253	Metoclopramide	
254	Mycophenolate	
255	Carisoprodol	
256	Calcitriol	
257	Linaclotide	
258	Anastrozole	
259	Dapagliflozin	
260	Exenatide	
261	Ziprasidone	
262	Calcium	
263	Epinephrine	
264	Torsemide	
265	Insulin Degludec	
266	Alfuzosin	

Rank	GENERIC	BRAND
267	Sotalol	
268	Bisoprolol	
269	Quinapril	
270	Olopatadine	
271	Ketorolac	
272	Methylcellulose	
273	Ranolazine	
274	Lurasidone	
275	Pancrelipase	
276	Dutasteride	
277	Bumetanide	
278	Ofloxacin	
279	Rabeprazole	
280	Triazolam	
281	Dorzolamide	
282	Tadalafil	
283	Solifenacin	
284	Ethinyl Estradiol + Norgestrel	
285	Vilazodone	
286	Chlorhexidine	
287	Sennosides	
288	Buprenorphine + Naloxone	
289	Flecainide	
290	Niacin	
291	Indomethacin	
292	Hydrochlorothiazide + Olmesartan	
293	Tretinoin	
294	Conjugated Estrogens + Medroxyprogesterone	
295	Atenolol + Chlorthalidone	
296	Haloperidol	

Rank	GENERIC	BRAND
297	Azelastine	
298	Ezetimibe + Simvastatin	
299	Enoxaparin	
300	Betamethasone + Clotrimazole	

By Classification (Top 300)

Fill out the brand names of the following generic medications

#	GENERIC	BRAND
1	Dutasteride	
2	Finasteride	
3	Mesalamine	
4	Tretinoin	
5	Tizanidine	
6	Alfuzosin	
7	Brimonidine tartrate	
8	Doxazosin	
9	Prazosin	
10	Tamsulosin	
11	Terazosin	
12	Hydroxychloroquine	
13	Acetaminophen	
14	Menthol	
15	Acetaminophen + Hydrocodone	
16	Fentanyl	
17	Hydrocodone Bitartrate	
18	Hydromorphone	
19	Morphine Sulfate	
20	Oxycodone	
21	Tramadol	
22	Acetaminophen + Butalbital	
23	Epinephrine Auto-Injector	
24	Testosterone	
25	Irbesartan	
26	Losartan	
27	Olmesartan	
28	Telmisartan	

#	GENERIC	BRAND
29	Valsartan	
30	Benazepril	
31	Enalapril	
32	Lisinopril	
33	Quinapril	
34	Ramipril	
35	Calcium	
36	Magnesium Oxide	
37	Ranolazine	
38	Amiodarone	
39	Digoxin	
40	Flecainide	
41	Sotalol	
42	Amoxicillin	
43	Amoxicillin + Clavulanate	
44	Bacitracin + Neomycin + Polymyxin B	
45	Cefdinir	
46	Cephalexin	
47	Chlorhexidine	
48	Clindamycin	
49	Mupirocin	
50	Nitrofurantoin	
51	Sulfamethoxazole + Trimethoprim	
52	Ciprofloxacin Oral	
53	Levofloxacin	
54	Azithromycin	
55	Erythromycin	
56	Penicillin VK	
57	Ofloxacin	
58	Doxycycline	
59	Minocycline	
60	Dicyclomine	

#	GENERIC	BRAND
61	Solifenacin	
62	Tolterodine	
63	Apixaban	
64	Enoxaparin	
65	Warfarin	
66	Rivaroxaban	
67	Carbamazepine	
68	Divalproex	
69	Gabapentin	
70	Lamotrigine	
71	Levetiracetam	
72	Oxcarbazepine	
73	Phenytoin	
74	Primidone	
75	Topiramate	
76	Pregabalin	
77	Trazodone	
78	Amitriptyline	
79	Doxepin	
80	Nortriptyline	
81	Bupropion	
82	Mirtazapine	
83	Venlafaxine	
84	Citalopram	
85	Escitalopram	
86	Fluoxetine	
87	Paroxetine	
88	Sertraline	
89	Vilazodone	
90	Metformin + Sitagliptin	
91	Sitagliptin	
92	Insulin Degludec	

#	GENERIC	BRAND
93	Insulin Detemir	
94	Insulin Glargine	
95	Insulin Aspart	
96	Insulin Lispro	
97	Insulin Human	
98	Empagliflozin	
99	Glimepiride	
100	Glipizide	
101	Glyburide	
102	Pioglitazone	
103	Ondansetron	
104	Metoclopramide	
105	Fluconazole	
106	Ketoconazole Topical	
107	Nystatin	
108	Metronidazole	
109	Bimatoprost	
110	Dorzolamide	
111	Dorzolamide + Timolol	
112	Travoprost	
113	Timolol	
114	Azelastine	
115	Cetirizine	
116	Fexofenadine	
117	Levocetirizine	
118	Loratadine	
119	Olopatadine	
120	Naphazoline + Pheniramine	
121	Diphenhydramine	
122	Hydroxyzine	
123	Meclizine	
124	Promethazine	

#	GENERIC	BRAND
125	Ezetimibe	
126	Ezetimibe + Simvastatin	
127	Niacin	
128	Omega-3 Fatty Acid Ethyl Esters	
129	Fenofibrate	
130	Gemfibrozil	
131	Atorvastatin	
132	Lovastatin	
133	Pravastatin	
134	Rosuvastatin	
135	Simvastatin	
136	Lithium	
137	Rizatriptan	
138	Sumatriptan	
139	Tamoxifen	
140	Anastrozole	
141	Carbidopa + Levodopa	
142	Benztropine	
143	Pramipexole	
144	Ropinirole	
145	Clopidogrel	
146	Aspirin	
147	Haloperidol	
148	Lurasidone	
149	Ziprasidone	
150	Aripiprazole	
151	Olanzapine	
152	Quetiapine	
153	Risperidone	
154	Oxybutynin	
155	Benzonatate	
156	Guaifenesin + Pseudoephedrine + Codeine	

#	GENERIC	BRAND
157	Acyclovir	
158	Oseltamivir	
159	Valacyclovir	
160	Clonazepam	
161	Alprazolam	
162	Buspirone	
163	Lorazepam	
164	Diazepam	
165	Mirabegron	
166	Atenolol	
167	Bisoprolol	
168	Carvedilol	
169	Labetalol	
170	Metoprolol	
171	Nebivolol	
172	Propranolol	
173	Atenolol + Chlorthalidone	
174	Metformin	
175	Alendronate	
176	Albuterol	
177	Ipratropium Bromide	
178	Tiotropium	
179	Amlodipine	
180	Diltiazem	
181	Nifedipine	
182	Verapamil	
183	Amlodipine + Benazepril	
184	Donepezil	
185	Atomoxetine	
186	Dexmethylphenidate Hydrochloride	
187	Dextroamphetamine + Amphetamine	
188	Lisdexamfetamine	

#	GENERIC	BRAND
189	Methylphenidate	
190	Phentermine	
191	Desogestrel + Ethinyl Estradiol	
192	Drospirenone + Ethinyl estradiol	
193	Ethinyl Estradiol + Etonogestrel	
194	Ethinyl Estradiol + Levonorgestrel	
195	Ethinyl Estradiol + Norethindrone	
196	Ethinyl Estradiol + Norgestimate	
197	Ethinyl Estradiol + Norgestrel	
198	Norethindrone	
199	Beclomethasone Dipropionate	
200	Budesonide	
201	Clobetasol	
202	Hydrocortisone Topical	
203	Mometasone Nasal	
204	Prednisone	
205	Triamcinolone Topical	
206	Fluticasone + Salmeterol	
207	Betamethasone Dipropionate + Clotrimazole	
208	Methylprednisolone	
209	Sodium Chloride	
210	Linagliptin	
211	Bumetanide	
212	Furosemide	
213	Torsemide	
214	HCTZ + Triamterene	
215	Spironolactone	
216	Chlorthalidone	
217	Hydrochlorothiazide (HCTZ)	
218	HCTZ + Losartan	
219	HCTZ + Olmesartan	
220	HCTZ + Valsartan	

#	GENERIC	BRAND
221	Hydrochlorothiazide (HCTZ) + Lisinopril	
222	Adalimumab	
223	Potassium Chloride	
224	Estradiol oral	
225	Estrogens, Conjugated	
226	Guaifenesin	
227	Sucralfate	
228	Linaclotide	
229	Dulaglutide	
230	Exenatide	
231	Liraglutide	
232	Prednisolone Oral	
233	Famotidine	
234	Ranitidine	
235	Emtricitabine	
236	Conjugated Estrogens + Medroxyprogesterone	
237	Mycophenolate	
238	Methotrexate	
239	Cyclosporine	
240	Fluticasone	
241	Ferrous Sulfate	
242	Docusate Sodium	
243	Methylcellulose	
244	Polyethylene Glycol 3350	
245	Sennosides	
246	Montelukast	
247	Lidocaine Patch	
248	Isosorbide Mononitrate	
249	Nitroglycerin	
250	Memantine	
251	Celecoxib	
252	Diclofenac Sodium	

#	GENERIC	BRAND
253	Ibuprofen	
254	Indomethacin	
255	Ketorolac	
256	Meloxicam	
257	Naproxen	
258	Buprenorphine + Naloxone	
259	Sodium Fluoride	
260	Pancrelipase	
261	Hydralazine	
262	Sildenafil	
263	Tadalafil	
264	Medroxyprogesterone	
265	Progesterone	
266	Latanoprost	
267	Dexlansoprazole	
268	Esomeprazole	
269	Lansoprazole	
270	Omeprazole	
271	Rabeprazole	
272	Pantoprazole	
273	Albuterol Sulfate + Ipratropium Bromide	
274	Budesonide + Formoterol	
275	Formoterol + Mometasone	
276	Eszopiclone	
277	Temazepam	
278	Triazolam	
279	Zolpidem	
280	Desvenlafaxine	
281	Duloxetine	
282	Baclofen	
283	Carisoprodol	
284	Cyclobenzaprine	

#	GENERIC	BRAND
285	Methocarbamol	
286	Canagliflozin	
287	Dapagliflozin	
288	Levothyroxine	
289	Liothyronine	
290	Methimazole	
291	Thyroid	
292	Colchicine	
293	Calcitriol	
294	Calcium + Cholecalciferol	
295	Ergocalciferol	
296	Cyanocobalamin	
297	Folic Acid	
298	Allopurinol	
299	Clonidine	
300	Guanfacine	

By Brand (Top 300)

Fill out the generic names of the following brand medications

#	BRAND	GENERIC
1	Abilify	
2	Accupril	
3	Aciphex	
4	Actos	
5	Adderall	
6	Adipex-P, Lomaira	
7	Advair Diskus, Advair HFA	
8	Aldactone	
9	Allegra	
10	Alphagan P	
11	Altace	
12	Amaryl	
13	Ambien	
14	Amoxil	
15	Anaprox	
16	Androgel, Androderm	
17	Antivert, Bonine, Dramamine	
18	Apresoline	
19	Apri, Cyclessa, Enskyce, Viorele	
20	Aricept	
21	Arimidex	
22	Armour Thyroid	
23	Asacol	
24	Astelin	
25	Atarax, Vistaril	
26	Ativan	
27	Atrovent HFA	
28	Augmentin	

#	BRAND	GENERIC
29	Avapro	
30	Avodart	
31	Bactrim	
32	Bactroban	
33	Benadryl	
34	Bengay Cold Therapy	
35	Benicar	
36	Benicar HCT	
37	Bentyl	
38	Betapace, Sorine	
39	Bumex	
40	Buspar	
41	Byetta, Bydureon	
42	Bystolic	
43	Calan SR	
44	Carafate	
45	Cardizem	
46	Cardura	
47	Catapres	
48	Celebrex	
49	Celexa	
50	CellCept	
51	Cheratussin DAC	
52	Cialis	
53	Cipro	
54	Citrucel	
55	Claritin	
56	Cleocin	
57	Cogentin	
58	Colace	
59	Colcrys	
60	Combivent Respimat	

#	BRAND	GENERIC
61	Cordarone	
62	Coreg	
63	Cortisone	
64	Cosopt	
65	Coumadin	
66	Cozaar	
67	Creon	
68	Crestor	
69	Cryselle	
70	Cymbalta	
71	Cytomel	
72	Deltasone	
73	Demadex	
74	Depakote	
75	Desyrel	
76	Detrol LA	
77	Dexilant	
78	Diflucan	
79	Dilantin	
80	Dilaudid	
81	Diovan	
82	Diovan HCT	
83	Ditropan	
84	Drenaclick, EpiPen	
85	Dulera	
86	Duragesic Patch	
87	Dyazide	
88	Dynacin, Minocin	
89	Ecotrin	
90	Effexor	
91	Elavil	
92	Eliquis	

#	BRAND	GENERIC
93	Emtriva	
94	Errin, Heather	
95	Erythrocin	
96	Estrace	
97	Farxiga	
98	Feosol	
99	Flagyl	
100	Flexeril	
101	Flomax	
102	Flonase	
103	Focalin	
104	Folate, Folvite	
105	Fosamax	
106	Geodon	
107	Glucophage	
108	Glucotrol	
109	Golytely	
110	Halcion	
111	Haldol	
112	Humalog	
113	Humira	
114	Humulin R, Novolin R	
115	Hygroton, Thalitone	
116	Hytrin	
117	Hyzaar	
118	Imdur	
119	Imitrex	
120	Impoyz, Temovate	
121	Inderal	
122	Indocin, Tivorbex	
123	Intuniv	
124	Invokana	

#	BRAND	GENERIC
125	Janumet XR	
126	Januvia	
127	Jardiance	
128	Keflex	
129	Kenalog	
130	Keppra	
131	Klonopin	
132	Klor-Con	
133	Lamictal	
134	Lanoxin	
135	Lantus	
136	Lasix	
137	Latuda	
138	Levaquin	
139	Levemir	
140	Lexapro	
141	Lidoderm	
142	Linzess	
143	Lioresal	
144	Lipitor	
145	Lithobid	
146	Lopid	
147	Lotensin	
148	Lotrel	
149	Lotrisone	
150	Lovaza	
151	Lovenox	
152	Lumigan	
153	Lunesta	
154	Lyrica	
155	Macrobid	
156	Mag-Ox 400	

#	BRAND	GENERIC
157	Maxalt	
158	Medrol	
159	Mevacor	
160	Micardis	
161	Micronase, Diabeta	
162	Microzide	
163	Minipress, Prazo, Prazin	
164	Mirapex	
165	Mobic	
166	Motrin, Advil	
167	MS Contin, Avinza, Kadian	
168	Mucinex	
169	Mycostatin, Nystop	
170	Myrbetriq	
171	Mysoline	
172	Namenda	
173	Naphcon-A, Opcon-A, Visine-A	
174	Nasonex	
175	Necon 777	
176	Neoral, Sandimmune, Gengraf	
177	Neosporin	
178	Neurontin	
179	Nexium	
180	Niaspan, Slo-Niacin	
181	Nitrostat, Minitran	
182	Nizoral	
183	Norco, Vicodin, Lorcet	
184	Normodyne	
185	Norvasc	
186	Novolog	
187	NuvaRing	
188	Ocean, Ayr Saline	

#	BRAND	GENERIC
189	Ocuflox	
190	Omnicef	
191	Orapred, Prelone	
192	Os-Cal Ultra	
193	OxyContin	
194	Pamelor	
195	Patanol, Pataday	
196	Paxil	
197	Penicillin V	
198	Pepcid	
199	Peridex, PerioGard	
200	Phenergan	
201	Phrenilin Forte	
202	Plaquenil	
203	Plavix	
204	Pravachol	
205	Premarin	
206	Prempro	
207	Prevacid	
208	PreviDent	
209	Prilosec	
210	Prinivil, Zestril	
211	Pristiq	
212	Proair HFA, Proventil HFA, Ventolin HFA	
213	Procardia, Adalat	
214	Prometrium	
215	Proscar, Propecia	
216	Protonix	
217	Provera, Depo-Provera	
218	Prozac	
219	Pulmicort Flexhaler	
220	Qvar	

#	BRAND	GENERIC
221	Ranexa	
222	Reglan	
223	Remeron	
224	Requip	
225	Restoril	
226	Retin A	
227	Risperdal	
228	Ritalin, Concerta	
229	Robaxin	
230	Rocaltrol	
231	Senna, Senokot	
232	Seroquel	
233	Sinemet	
234	Sinequan, Silenor	
235	Singulair	
236	Soltamox	
237	Soma	
238	Spiriva Handihaler	
239	Strattera	
240	Suboxone	
241	Symbicort	
242	Synthroid	
243	Tambacor	
244	Tamiflu	
245	Tapazole	
246	Tegretol	
247	Tenoretic	
248	Tenormin	
249	Tessalon Perles	
250	Timoptic	
251	Topamax	
252	Toprol XL, Lopressor	

#	BRAND	GENERIC
253	Toradol	
254	Tradjenta	
255	Travatan Z	
256	Tresiba	
257	Trexall	
258	Tricor, Trilipix	
259	Trileptal	
260	Trinessa-28, Ortho Tri-Cyclen	
261	Trulicity	
262	Trusopt	
263	Tums	
264	Twirla	
265	Tylenol	
266	Ultram	
267	Uroxatral	
268	Valium	
269	Valtrex	
270	Vasotec	
271	Vesicare	
272	Viagra, Revatio	
273	Vibramycin	
274	Victoza, Saxenda	
275	Viibryd	
276	Vitamin B12	
277	Vitamin D	
278	Voltaren	
279	Vytorin	
280	Vyvanse	
281	Wellbutrin, Zyban	
282	Xalatan	
283	Xanax	
284	Xarelto	

#	BRAND	GENERIC
285	Xyzal	
286	Yaz	
287	Zanaflex	
288	Zantac	
289	Zebeta	
290	Zestoretic	
291	Zetia	
292	Zocor	
293	Zofran	
294	Zohydro ER	
295	Zoloft	
296	Zovirax	
297	Z-Pak, Zithromax	
298	Zyloprim	
299	Zyprexa	
300	Zyrtec	

Extra Practice 100 Medications

Fill out the brand names of the following generic medications

#	GENERIC	BRAND
1	Adapalene	
2	Abacavir + Lamivudine	
3	Acetaminophen + Codeine	
4	Acetaminophen + Oxycodone	
5	Acetaminophen + Tramadol	
6	Aliskiren	
7	Amlodipine + Olmesartan	
8	Amlodipine + Valsartan	
9	Atazanavir	
10	Azathioprine	
11	Benzoyl Peroxide + Clindamycin	
12	Butalbital + Caffeine + Acetaminophen	
13	Butalbital + Caffeine + Aspirin	
14	Candesartan	
15	Candesartan + HCTZ	
16	Captopril	
17	Cefaclor	
18	Cefazolin	
19	Cefprozil	
20	Cefuroxime	
21	Cinacalcet	
22	Ciprofloxacin + Dexamethasone Otic (Ear Drop)	
23	Clarithromycin	
24	Clobazam	
25	Clorazepate	
26	Colesevelam	
27	Dabigatran	
28	Dexamethasone	

#	GENERIC	BRAND
29	Diphenoxylate and Atropine	
30	Efavirenz	
31	Eletriptan	
32	Elmisartan + HCTZ	
33	Emtricitabine + Tenofovir	
34	Entecavir	
35	Etodolac	
36	Febuxostat	
37	Felodipine	
38	Fexofenadine + Pseudoephedrine	
39	Fluocinonide Topical	
40	Fluvoxamine	
41	Fosinopril	
42	Gatifloxacin	
43	Hepatitis A Vaccine	
44	Hepatitis B Vaccine	
45	Herpes Zoster Vaccine	
46	Human Papillomavirus Vaccine	
47	Hydrocodone + Ibuprofen	
48	Ibandronate	
49	Imiquimod	
50	Influenza Vaccine	
51	Insulin Aspart Protamine (70%), Aspart (30%)	
52	Insulin Glulisine	
53	Insulin NPH	
54	Insulin NPH (70%),	
55	Irbesartan + HCTZ	
56	Isotretinoin	
57	Lacosamide	
58	Levalbuterol	
59	Loteprednol	
60	Lubiprostone	

#	GENERIC	BRAND
61	Maraviroc	
62	Measles, Mumps, Rubella Vaccine	
63	Meningococcal Vaccine	
64	Meperidine	
65	Methadone	
66	Methylprednisolone	
67	Moxifloxacin	
68	Nabumetone	
69	Nateglinide	
70	Perindopril	
71	Phenazopyridine	
72	Phenobarbital	
73	Piroxicam	
74	Pneumococcal Vaccine	
75	Polio Vaccine	
76	Prochlorperazine	
77	Raloxifene	
78	Raltegravir	
79	Ramelteon	
80	Regular (30%)	
81	Repaglinide	
82	Rifaximin	
83	Risedronate	
84	Rosiglitazone	
85	Rotavirus Vaccine	
86	Sacubitril + Valsartan	
87	Saxagliptin	
88	Scopolamine	
89	Sevelamer carbonate	
90	Tacrolimus	
91	Tdap (Tetanus, Diphtheria, Pertussis)	
92	Terbinafine	

#	GENERIC	BRAND
93	Ticagrelor	
94	Tobramycin	
95	Tropium	
96	Vancomycin	
97	Vardenafil	
98	Varenicline	
99	Zaleplon	
100	Zolmitriptan	

WAYS TO GET A PHARMACY TECH LICENSE

T here are many ways to go about getting a pharmacy technician license, which allows you to legally work at a variety of places such as hospitals, home infusion pharmacies, community pharmacies and other healthcare settings. Depending on the option you choose, it could easily cost $10–15k or more. Less expensive alternatives are available and will be discussed later in this chapter.

Monetary investment aside, the time component is another important factor worth considering. Traditional routes normally take 9–15 months to complete, and they could easily be found with a quick search on Google/the internet. Although shorter online programs are available, they are not as popular due to their lack of hands-on experience. What many students do know is the fact that hands-on experience can easily be obtained by working or volunteering as a pharmacy clerk.

In order to get a pharmacy technician license, you must be a high school graduate or have a general education development (GED) certificate equivalent. In addition, you also need to fulfill the pharmacy technician training requirement, which can be achieved in a few different ways.

The following are the five common ways to obtain a pharmacy technician license:

1. Complete an Associate Degree in Pharmacy Technology;

2. Complete a pharmacy technician training program accredited by the American Society of Health-System Pharmacists (ASHP);

3. Graduate from a school of pharmacy accredited by the Accreditation Council for Pharmacy Education (ACPE).

4. Pass the PTCB (Pharmacy Technician Certification Board) exam commonly known as the PTCE

5. Pass the ExCPT exam by the National Healthcare Association

A less common way that many students are unaware of is through an employer's training program that requires a minimum of 240 hours of instructions. In the past, whenever people asked me about the best way to get a pharmacy technician license, I would suggest they go with the least expensive option they could find. Nowadays, I would recommend that they get paid in the process of accomplishing that goal. The employer's training program is one of them and the exact steps on how to do that, specifically in California, are discussed later in this chapter. The other method is by passing the PTCE or ExCPT exam, which allows you to apply for the license afterward.

For those in the military, there is a special training provided by a branch of the federal armed services that will prepare you to get a pharmacy technician license. All you need to do is to submit to the board of pharmacy a copy of your DD214 documenting evidence of the training you have received.

How to Get a Pharmacy Tech License in California without Paying $15k or MORE

———— ❧ ————

U
nknown to many is the process of becoming a licensed pharmacy technician in the State of California while getting paid for doing so. I was not aware of this somewhat obscure fact for years, and it is easy to understand why it has been kept as such by many private institutions. There might be a similar path to obtain the license in other states, and the best place to look for that information is probably from the Board of Pharmacy website.

I will outline a Three-Steps Process to obtain a pharmacy technician license in California without going through the conventional pharmacy program that could cost $10 –15k or more. However, before you get started, it is critical to note that you must be a high school graduate or have a general education development (GED) certificate equivalent.

STEP 1: Start working and getting paid as a clerk at your local retail pharmacy. Retail pharmacy refers to any chain pharmacy (such as CVS, Walgreens, or Walmart), independent pharmacy, or compounding pharmacy. A license is not required to work as a clerk.

STEP 2: After completing 240 hours (1.5 to two months if you work an average of 30-40 hours per week), download the "PHARMACY TECHNICIAN APPLICATION" form from the California Board of Pharmacy website or via the following link: https://www.pharmacy.ca.gov/forms/tch_app_pkt.pdf

STEP 3: Follow the detailed instructions provided on the form. Part 6 on page two of the instruction lists four possible documents you could provide. However, the only applicable option here is **(A) Any other course that provides a training**

period of at least 240 hours of instruction as specified in Title 16 California Code of Regulation section 1793.6(c). Make sure to get the pharmacist's signature on page four, and you must also attach a pharmacist's business card with a license number along with the application. Fill out the application completely and submit it with the required fees.

I know that might sound really simple, and the truth is it really is that simple.

Get Paid Preparing for the PTCE

———— ✺ ————

To be eligible for the PTCE, a candidate must complete one of the following two pathways:

- **Pathway 1**: A PTCB-Recognized Education/Training Program (or completion within 60 days). Candidates choose from more than 1,400 recognized programs.

- **Pathway 2**: Equivalent work experience as a pharmacy technician (min. 500 hours). This alternative secondary path serves experienced technicians who were not in a position to attend a PTCB-recognized program. PTCB accepts work experience across pharmacy practice settings that pertains to certain knowledge requirements.

Pathway 2 is how you can avoid taking the traditional training program that could cost $15k or more depending on where you take them. It is also how you get paid while making yourself eligible to take the PTCE (by meeting the 500 hours of work experience requirement) and get the CPhT credential once you pass.

Get Paid Preparing for the ExCPT Exam

To be eligible to sit for the ExCPT Pharmacy Technician Exam, you must:

1. Have a high school diploma or the equivalent such as the General Education Development test (GED)

2. Successfully complete a training program or have relevant work experience as described below:

   a. Successfully complete an employer-based training program that:

      i. is recognized by the Board of Pharmacy of the state in which the candidate completes the training program; or

      ii. has been verified by the candidate's employer to provide academic preparation, including technical skills and knowledge, sufficient to prepare the candidate to adequately perform the duties of an entry-level pharmacy technician.

   b. Work Experience - Candidates must have completed at least 1200 hours of supervised pharmacy-related work experience within any one (1) year of the past three (3) years.

Option 2b is how you can avoid taking the traditional training program. It is also how you get paid while making yourself eligible to take the ExCPT exam (by meeting the 1200 hours of supervised pharmacy-related work experience) and get the CPhT credential once you pass. Unless you plan to change your career, it doesn't make a lot of sense to pay $10k or more for a program when you can make $15k or more while preparing for the same examination.

ANSWERS

By Rank (Top 300)

Rank	GENERIC	BRAND
1	Lisinopril	Prinivil, Zestril
2	Atorvastatin	Lipitor
3	Levothyroxine	Synthroid
4	Metformin Hydrochloride	Glucophage
5	Amlodipine	Norvasc
6	Metoprolol	Toprol XL, Lopressor
7	Omeprazole	Prilosec
8	Simvastatin	Zocor
9	Losartan Potassium	Cozaar
10	Albuterol	Proair HFA, Proventil HFA, Ventolin HFA
11	Gabapentin	Neurontin
12	Hydrochlorothiazide	Benicar HCT
13	Acetaminophen; Hydrocodone Bitartrate	Norco, Vicodin, Lorcet
14	Sertraline Hydrochloride	Zoloft
15	Fluticasone	Flonase, Veramyst, Flovent HFA, Arnuity Ellipta, Flovent Diskus
16	Montelukast	Singulair
17	Furosemide	Lasix
18	Amoxicillin	Amoxil
19	Pantoprazole Sodium	Protonix

Rank	GENERIC	BRAND
20	Escitalopram Oxalate	Lexapro
21	Alprazolam	Xanax
22	Prednisone	Deltasone
23	Bupropion	Wellbutrin, Zyban
24	Pravastatin Sodium	Pravachol
25	Acetaminophen	Tylenol
26	Citalopram	Celexa
27	Dextroamphetamine; Dextroamphetamine Saccharate; Amphetamine; Amphetamine Aspartate	Adderall
28	Ibuprofen	Motrin, Advil
29	Carvedilol	Coreg
30	Trazodone Hydrochloride	Desyrel
31	Fluoxetine Hydrochloride	Prozac
32	Tramadol Hydrochloride	Ultram
33	Insulin Glargine	Lantus
34	Clonazepam	Klonopin
35	Tamsulosin Hydrochloride	Flomax
36	Atenolol	Tenormin
37	Potassium	Klor-Con
38	Meloxicam	Mobic
39	Rosuvastatin	Crestor
40	Clopidogrel Bisulfate	Plavix
41	Propranolol Hydrochloride	Inderal
42	Aspirin	Ecotrin
43	Cyclobenzaprine	Flexeril
44	Hydrochlorothiazide; Lisinopril	Dyazide, Maxzide
45	Glipizide	Glucotrol
46	Duloxetine	Cymbalta
47	Methylphenidate	Ritalin, Concerta
48	Ranitidine	Zantac
49	Venlafaxine	Effexor
50	Zolpidem Tartrate	Ambien, Ambien CR, Intermezzo

Rank	GENERIC	BRAND
51	Warfarin	Coumadin
52	Oxycodone	OxyContin
53	Ethinyl Estradiol; Norethindrone	Necon 777
54	Allopurinol	Zyloprim
55	Ergocalciferol	Vitamin D
56	Insulin Aspart	Novolog
57	Azithromycin	Z-Pak, Zithromax
58	Metronidazole	Flagyl
59	Loratadine	Claritin, Alavert
60	Lorazepam	Ativan
61	Estradiol	Estrace
62	Ethinyl Estradiol; Norgestimate	Trinessa-28, Ortho Tri-Cyclen, Ortho Tri-Cyclen Lo
63	Lamotrigine	Lamictal
64	Glimepiride	Amaryl
65	Fluticasone Propionate; Salmeterol Xinafoate	Advair Diskus, Advair HFA
66	Cetirizine	Zyrtec
67	Hydrochlorothiazide; Losartan Potassium	Diovan HCT
68	Paroxetine	Paxil
69	Spironolactone	Aldactone
70	Fenofibrate	Tricor, Trilipix, Antara, Fenoglide, Lipofen, Lofibra, Trilipix
71	Naproxen	Anaprox
72	Pregabalin	Lyrica
73	Insulin Human	Humulin R, Novolin R
74	Budesonide; Formoterol	Symbicort
75	Diltiazem Hydrochloride	Cardizem, Cartia XT
76	Quetiapine Fumarate	Seroquel
77	Topiramate	Topamax
78	Bacitracin; Neomycin; Polymyxin B	Neosporin
79	Clonidine	Catapres
80	Buspirone Hydrochloride	Buspar

Rank	GENERIC	BRAND
81	Latanoprost	Xalatan
82	Tiotropium	Spiriva Handihaler
83	Ondansetron	Zofran
84	Lovastatin	Mevacor, Altoprev
85	Valsartan	Diovan
86	Finasteride	Proscar, Propecia
87	Amitriptyline	Elavil
88	Esomeprazole	Nexium
89	Tizanidine	Zanaflex
90	Alendronate Sodium	Fosamax
91	Lisdexamfetamine Dimesylate	Vyvanse
92	Ferrous Sulfate	Feosol, Fer-In-Sol
93	Apixaban	Eliquis
94	Diclofenac	Voltaren, Cambia, Zipsor, Zorvolex
95	Sitagliptin Phosphate	Januvia
96	Folic Acid	Folate, Folvite
97	Sumatriptan	Imitrex
98	Drospirenone; Ethinyl Estradiol	Yaz
99	Hydroxyzine	Atarax, Vistaril
100	Oxybutynin	Ditropan
101	Hydrochlorothiazide; Triamterene	Microzide
102	Cephalexin	Keflex
103	Triamcinolone	Kenalog, Trianex, Triacet, Nasacort AQ
104	Benazepril Hydrochloride	Lotensin
105	Hydralazine Hydrochloride	Hyzaar
106	Celecoxib	Celebrex
107	Ciprofloxacin	Cipro
108	Ropinirole Hydrochloride	Requip
109	Rivaroxaban	Xarelto
110	Levetiracetam	Keppra
111	Isosorbide Mononitrate	Imdur
112	Aripiprazole	Abilify

Rank	GENERIC	BRAND
113	Doxycycline	Vibramycin
114	Insulin Detemir	Levemir
115	Famotidine	Pepcid
116	Amoxicillin; Clavulanate Potassium	Augmentin
117	Methotrexate	Trexall
118	Hydrocodone Bitartrate	Zohydro ER, Hysingla ER, Vantrela ER
119	Mirtazapine	Remeron
120	Nifedipine	Procardia, Adalat
121	Sulfamethoxazole; Trimethoprim	Bactrim
122	Enalapril Maleate	Vasotec
123	Docusate	Colace
124	Insulin Lispro	Humalog
125	Pioglitazone	Actos
126	Divalproex Sodium	Depakote, Depakote ER
127	Donepezil Hydrochloride	Aricept
128	Hydroxychloroquine Sulfate	Plaquenil
129	Prednisolone	Orapred, Prelone, Pediapred
130	Thyroid	Armour Thyroid
131	Guanfacine	Intuniv
132	Testosterone	Androgel, Androderm
133	Hydrochlorothiazide; Valsartan	Zestoretic
134	Ramipril	Altace
135	Diazepam	Valium
136	Ethinyl Estradiol; Levonorgestrel	Twirla
137	Clindamycin	Cleocin
138	Gemfibrozil	Lopid
139	Metformin Hydrochloride; Sitagliptin Phosphate	Janumet XR
140	Baclofen	Lioresal
141	Norethindrone	Errin, Heather, Camila
142	Temazepam	Restoril
143	Nitroglycerin	Nitrostat, Minitran
144	Nebivolol Hydrochloride	Bystolic

Rank	GENERIC	BRAND
145	Verapamil Hydrochloride	Calan SR
146	Timolol	Timoptic
147	Promethazine Hydrochloride	Phenergan
148	Benzonatate	Tessalon Perles
149	Memantine Hydrochloride	Namenda
150	Doxazosin Mesylate	Cardura, Cardura-XL
151	Ezetimibe	Zetia
152	Valacyclovir	Valtrex
153	Beclomethasone	Qvar
154	Hydrocortisone	Cortisone
155	Morphine	MS Contin, Avinza, Kadian
156	Risperidone	Risperdal
157	Methylprednisolone	Medrol
158	Omega-3-acid Ethyl Esters	Lovaza
159	Oseltamivir Phosphate	Tamiflu
160	Amlodipine Besylate; Benazepril Hydrochloride	Lotrel
161	Meclizine Hydrochloride	Antivert, Bonine, Dramamine
162	Polyethylene Glycol 3350	Golytely
163	Liraglutide	Victoza, Saxenda
164	Desogestrel; Ethinyl Estradiol	Apri, Cyclessa, Enskyce, Viorele
165	Levofloxacin	Levaquin
166	Acyclovir	Zovirax
167	Brimonidine Tartrate	Alphagan P
168	Digoxin	Lanoxin
169	Adalimumab	Humira
170	Cyanocobalamin	Vitamin B12
171	Magnesium	Mag-Ox 400
172	Albuterol Sulfate; Ipratropium Bromide	Combivent Respimat
173	Chlorthalidone	Hygroton, Thalitone
174	Glyburide	Micronase, Diabeta
175	Levocetirizine Dihydrochloride	Xyzal
176	Carbamazepine	Tegretol
177	Ethinyl Estradiol; Etonogestrel	NuvaRing

Rank	GENERIC	BRAND
178	Methocarbamol	Robaxin
179	Pramipexole Dihydrochloride	Mirapex
180	Lithium	Lithobid, Eskalith
181	Dicyclomine Hydrochloride	Bentyl
182	Fluconazole	Diflucan
183	Nortriptyline Hydrochloride	Pamelor
184	Carbidopa; Levodopa	Sinemet, Sinemet CR
185	Nitrofurantoin	Macrobid, Macrodantin
186	Mupirocin	Bactroban
187	Acetaminophen; Butalbital	Phrenilin Forte, Phrenilin, Bupap, Orbivan CF
188	Lansoprazole	Prevacid
189	Dexmethylphenidate Hydrochloride	Focalin
190	Budesonide	Pulmicort Flexhaler
191	Mirabegron	Myrbetriq
192	Canagliflozin	Invokana
193	Menthol	Bengay Cold Therapy, Icy Hot Naturals
194	Terazosin	Hytrin
195	Progesterone	Prometrium
196	Amiodarone Hydrochloride	Cordarone
197	Mometasone	Nasonex
198	Cefdinir	Omnicef
199	Atomoxetine Hydrochloride	Strattera
200	Linagliptin	Tradjenta
201	Colchicine	Colcrys
202	Dexlansoprazole	Dexilant
203	Naphazoline Hydrochloride; Pheniramine Maleate	Naphcon-A, Opcon-A, Visine-A
204	Rizatriptan Benzoate	Maxalt
205	Hydromorphone Hydrochloride	Dilaudid
206	Estrogens, Conjugated	Premarin
207	Oxcarbazepine	Trileptal
208	Lidocaine	Lidoderm
209	Clobetasol Propionate	Impoyz, Temovate

Rank	GENERIC	BRAND
210	Phentermine	Adipex-P, Lomaira
211	Labetalol	Normodyne
212	Travoprost	Travatan Z
213	Guaifenesin; Codeine Phosphate; Pseudoephedrine Hydrochloride	Cheratussin DAC, Virtussin DAC
214	Eszopiclone	Lunesta
215	Erythromycin	Erythrocin
216	Ipratropium	Atrovent HFA
217	Sildenafil	Viagra, Revatio
218	Sucralfate	Carafate
219	Ketoconazole	Nizoral
220	Irbesartan	Avapro
221	Phenytoin	Dilantin
222	Medroxyprogesterone Acetate	Provera, Depo-Provera
223	Olmesartan Medoxomil	Benicar
224	Emtricitabine	Emtriva
225	Sodium	Ocean, Ayr Saline
226	Benztropine Mesylate	Cogentin
227	Prazosin Hydrochloride	Minipress, Prazo, Prazin
228	Empagliflozin	Jardiance
229	Tolterodine Tartrate	Detrol LA
230	Nystatin	Mycostatin, Nyamyc, Nystop
231	Bimatoprost	Lumigan
232	Dulaglutide	Trulicity
233	Dorzolamide Hydrochloride; Timolol Maleate	Cosopt
234	Guaifenesin	Mucinex
235	Desvenlafaxine	Pristiq, Khedezla
236	Calcium; Cholecalciferol	Os-Cal Ultra, Caltrate 600 + D3
237	Minocycline Hydrochloride	Dynacin, Minocin, Solodyn
238	Primidone	Mysoline
239	Olanzapine	Zyprexa
240	Doxepin Hydrochloride	Sinequan, Silenor
241	Diphenhydramine Hydrochloride	Benadryl

Rank	GENERIC	BRAND
242	Penicillin V	Pen Vee K, Penicillin V
243	Formoterol Fumarate; Mometasone Furoate	Dulera
244	Methimazole	Tapazole
245	Fexofenadine Hydrochloride	Allegra
246	Mesalamine	Asacol
247	Sodium Fluoride	PreviDent
248	Cyclosporine	Neoral, Sandimmune, Gengraf
249	Telmisartan	Micardis
250	Fentanyl	Duragesic Patch, Lonsys
251	Tamoxifen Citrate	Soltamox
252	Liothyronine Sodium	Cytomel, Triostat
253	Metoclopramide Hydrochloride	Reglan
254	Mycophenolate Mofetil	CellCept, Myfortic
255	Carisoprodol	Soma
256	Calcitriol	Rocaltrol
257	Linaclotide	Linzess
258	Anastrozole	Arimidex
259	Dapagliflozin	Farxiga
260	Exenatide	Byetta, Bydureon
261	Ziprasidone	Geodon
262	Calcium	Tums, Oysco
263	Epinephrine	Drenaclick, Auvi-Q, EpiPen, EpiPen Jr
264	Torsemide	Demadex
265	Insulin Degludec	Tresiba
266	Alfuzosin Hydrochloride	Uroxatral
267	Sotalol Hydrochloride	Betapace, Sorine
268	Bisoprolol Fumarate	Zebeta
269	Quinapril	Accupril
270	Olopatadine	Patanol, Pataday
271	Ketorolac Tromethamine	Toradol
272	Methylcellulose (4000 Mpa.S)	Citrucel

Rank	GENERIC	BRAND
273	Ranolazine	Ranexa
274	Lurasidone Hydrochloride	Latuda
275	Pancrelipase Lipase; Pancrelipase Protease; Pancrelipase Amylase	Creon, Zenpep
276	Dutasteride	Avodart
277	Bumetanide	Bumex, Burinex
278	Ofloxacin	Ocuflox
279	Rabeprazole Sodium	Aciphex
280	Triazolam	Halcion
281	Dorzolamide Hydrochloride	Trusopt
282	Tadalafil	Cialis
283	Solifenacin Succinate	ritalin, Concerta
284	Ethinyl Estradiol; Norgestrel	Cryselle
285	Vilazodone Hydrochloride	Viibryd
286	Chlorhexidine	Peridex, PerioGard, PerioChip
287	Sennosides	Senna, Senokot
288	Buprenorphine; Naloxone	Suboxone, Bunavail, Zubsolv
289	Flecainide Acetate	Tambacor
290	Niacin	Niaspan, Slo-Niacin
291	Indomethacin	Indocin, Tivorbex
292	Hydrochlorothiazide; Olmesartan Medoxomil	Apresoline
293	Tretinoin	Retin A
294	Conjugated Estrogens; Medroxyprogesterone	Prempro
295	Atenolol; Chlorthalidone	Tenoretic
296	Haloperidol	Haldol
297	Azelastine Hydrochloride	Astelin, Astepro
298	Ezetimibe; Simvastatin	Vytorin
299	Enoxaparin Sodium	Lovenox
300	Betamethasone Dipropionate; Clotrimazole	Lotrisone

By Classification (Top 300)

#	GENERIC	BRAND	CLASS
1	Dutasteride	Avodart	5-Alpha-Reductase Inhibitor
2	Finasteride	Proscar, Propecia	5-Alpha-Reductase Inhibitor
3	Mesalamine	Asacol	5-Aminosalicylic Acid Derivatives
4	Tretinoin	Retin A	Acne Agent
5	Tizanidine	Zanaflex	Alpha 2 Adrenergic Agonist
6	Alfuzosin	Uroxatral	Alpha Blocker
7	Brimonidine tartrate	Alphagan P	Alpha Blocker
8	Doxazosin	Cardura, Cardura-XL	Alpha Blocker
9	Prazosin	Minipress, Prazo, Prazin	Alpha Blocker
10	Tamsulosin	Flomax	Alpha Blocker
11	Terazosin	Hytrin	Alpha Blocker
12	Hydroxychloroquine	Plaquenil	Aminoquinoline
13	Acetaminophen	Tylenol	Analgesic
14	Menthol	Bengay Cold Therapy, Icy Hot Naturals	Analgesic
15	Acetaminophen + Hydrocodone	Norco, Vicodin, Lorcet	Analgesic (Narcotic)
16	Fentanyl	Duragesic Patch, Lonsys	Analgesic (Opioid)
17	Hydrocodone Bitartrate	Zohydro ER, Hysingla ER, Vantrela ER	Analgesic (Opioid)
18	Hydromorphone	Dilaudid	Analgesic (Opioid)
19	Morphine Sulfate	MS Contin, Avinza, Kadian	Analgesic (Opioid)
20	Oxycodone	OxyContin	Analgesic (Opioid)
21	Tramadol	Ultram	Analgesic (Opioid)
22	Acetaminophen + Butalbital	Phrenilin Forte, Phrenilin, Bupap, Orbivan CF	Analgesic + Barbiturate Combo
23	Epinephrine Auto-Injector	Drenaclick, Auvi-Q, EpiPen, EpiPen Jr	Anaphylaxis Agent
24	Testosterone	Androgel, Androderm	Androgens
25	Irbesartan	Avapro	Angiotensin II Receptor Blocker
26	Losartan	Cozaar	Angiotensin II Receptor Blocker
27	Olmesartan	Benicar	Angiotensin II Receptor Blocker

#	GENERIC	BRAND	CLASS
28	Telmisartan	Micardis	Angiotensin II Receptor Blocker
29	Valsartan	Diovan	Angiotensin II Receptor Blocker
30	Benazepril	Lotensin	Angiotensin-converting enzyme (ACE) Inhibitor
31	Enalapril	Vasotec	Angiotensin-converting enzyme (ACE) Inhibitor
32	Lisinopril	Prinivil, Zestril	Angiotensin-converting enzyme (ACE) Inhibitor
33	Quinapril	Accupril	Angiotensin-converting enzyme (ACE) Inhibitor
34	Ramipril	Altace	Angiotensin-converting enzyme (ACE) Inhibitor
35	Calcium	Tums, Oysco	Antacid
36	Magnesium Oxide	Mag-Ox 400	Antacid, Electrolyte
37	Ranolazine	Ranexa	Antianginal, Non-nitrates
38	Amiodarone	Cordarone	Antiarrhythmic
39	Digoxin	Lanoxin	Antiarrhythmic
40	Flecainide	Tambacor	Antiarrhythmic
41	Sotalol	Betapace, Sorine	Antiarrhythmic
42	Amoxicillin	Amoxil	Antibiotic
43	Amoxicillin + Clavulanate	Augmentin	Antibiotic
44	Bacitracin + Neomycin + Polymyxin B	Neosporin	Antibiotic
45	Cefdinir	Omnicef	Antibiotic
46	Cephalexin	Keflex	Antibiotic
47	Chlorhexidine	Peridex, PerioGard, PerioChip	Antibiotic
48	Clindamycin	Cleocin	Antibiotic
49	Mupirocin	Bactroban	Antibiotic
50	Nitrofurantoin	Macrobid, Macrodantin	Antibiotic
51	Sulfamethoxazole + Trimethoprim	Bactrim	Antibiotic
52	Ciprofloxacin Oral	Cipro	Antibiotic (Fluoroquinolone)
53	Levofloxacin	Levaquin	Antibiotic (Fluoroquinolone)
54	Azithromycin	Z-Pak, Zithromax	Antibiotic (Macrolide)
55	Erythromycin	Erythrocin	Antibiotic (Macrolide)

#	GENERIC	BRAND	CLASS
56	Penicillin VK	Pen Vee K, Penicillin V	Antibiotic (Penicillin)
57	Ofloxacin	Ocuflox	Antibiotic (Quinolone)
58	Doxycycline	Vibramycin	Antibiotic (Tetracycline)
59	Minocycline	Dynacin, Minocin, Solodyn	Antibiotic (Tetracycline)
60	Dicyclomine	Bentyl	Anticholinergic
61	Solifenacin	Vesicare	Anticholinergic, Genitourinary
62	Tolterodine	Detrol LA	Anticholinergic, Genitourinary
63	Apixaban	Eliquis	Anticoagulant
64	Enoxaparin	Lovenox	Anticoagulant
65	Warfarin	Coumadin	Anticoagulant
66	Rivaroxaban	Xarelto	Anticoagulant, Factor Xa Inhibitor
67	Carbamazepine	Tegretol	Anticonvulsant
68	Divalproex	Depakote, Depakote ER	Anticonvulsant
69	Gabapentin	Neurontin	Anticonvulsant
70	Lamotrigine	Lamictal	Anticonvulsant
71	Levetiracetam	Keppra	Anticonvulsant
72	Oxcarbazepine	Trileptal	Anticonvulsant
73	Phenytoin	Dilantin	Anticonvulsant
74	Primidone	Mysoline	Anticonvulsant
75	Topiramate	Topamax	Anticonvulsant
76	Pregabalin	Lyrica	Anticonvulsant, Analgesic
77	Trazodone	Desyrel	Antidepressant
78	Amitriptyline	Elavil	Antidepressant (Tricyclic)
79	Doxepin	Sinequan, Silenor	Antidepressant (Tricyclic)
80	Nortriptyline	Pamelor	Antidepressant (Tricyclic)
81	Bupropion	Wellbutrin, Zyban	Antidepressant, Smoking Cessation Aids
82	Mirtazapine	Remeron	Antidepressant, SNRI
83	Venlafaxine	Effexor	Antidepressant, SNRI
84	Citalopram	Celexa	Antidepressant, SSRI
85	Escitalopram	Lexapro	Antidepressant, SSRI
86	Fluoxetine	Prozac	Antidepressant, SSRI

#	GENERIC	BRAND	CLASS
87	Paroxetine	Paxil	Antidepressant, SSRI
88	Sertraline	Zoloft	Antidepressant, SSRI
89	Vilazodone	Viibryd	Antidepressant, SSRI
90	Metformin + Sitagliptin	Janumet XR	Antidiabetic, Biguanides + Dipeptyl Peptidase-IV Inhibitor
91	Sitagliptin	Januvia	Antidiabetic, DPP4 Inhibitor
92	Insulin Degludec	Tresiba	Antidiabetic, Insulin, Long Acting
93	Insulin Detemir	Levemir	Antidiabetic, Insulin, Long Acting
94	Insulin Glargine	Lantus	Antidiabetic, Insulin, Long Acting
95	Insulin Aspart	Novolog	Antidiabetic, Insulin, Rapid Acting
96	Insulin Lispro	Humalog	Antidiabetic, Insulin, Rapid Acting
97	Insulin Human	Humulin R, Novolin R	Antidiabetic, Insulin, Short Acting
98	Empagliflozin	Jardiance	Antidiabetic, SGLT2 Inhibitor
99	Glimepiride	Amaryl	Antidiabetic, Sulfonylureas
100	Glipizide	Glucotrol	Antidiabetic, Sulfonylureas
101	Glyburide	Micronase, Diabeta	Antidiabetic, Sulfonylureas
102	Pioglitazone	Actos	Antidiabetic, Thiazolidinediones
103	Ondansetron	Zofran	Antiemetic
104	Metoclopramide	Reglan	Antiemetic, Prokinetic
105	Fluconazole	Diflucan	Antifungal
106	Ketoconazole Topical	Nizoral	Antifungal
107	Nystatin	Mycostatin, Nyamyc, Nystop	Antifungal
108	Metronidazole	Flagyl	Antifungal, Bacterial vaginosis, Intestinal infections
109	Bimatoprost	Lumigan	Antiglaucoma
110	Dorzolamide	Trusopt	Antiglaucoma
111	Dorzolamide + Timolol	Cosopt	Antiglaucoma
112	Travoprost	Travatan Z	Antiglaucoma
113	Timolol	Timoptic	Antiglaucoma, Beta Blocker
114	Azelastine	Astelin, Astepro	Antihistamine
115	Cetirizine	Zyrtec	Antihistamine
116	Fexofenadine	Allegra	Antihistamine
117	Levocetirizine	Xyzal	Antihistamine

#	GENERIC	BRAND	CLASS
118	Loratadine	Claritin, Alavert	Antihistamine
119	Olopatadine	Patanol, Pataday	Antihistamine
120	Naphazoline + Pheniramine	Naphcon-A, Opcon-A, Visine-A	Antihistamine + Decongestant
121	Diphenhydramine	Benadryl	Antihistamine, Antiemetic
122	Hydroxyzine	Atarax, Vistaril	Antihistamine, Antiemetic
123	Meclizine	Antivert, Bonine, Dramamine	Antihistamine, Antiemetic
124	Promethazine	Phenergan	Antihistamine, Antiemetic
125	Ezetimibe	Zetia	Antihyperlipidemic
126	Ezetimibe + Simvastatin	Vytorin	Antihyperlipidemic
127	Niacin	Niaspan, Slo-Niacin	Antihyperlipidemic
128	Omega-3 Fatty Acid Ethyl Esters	Lovaza	Antihyperlipidemic
129	Fenofibrate	Tricor, Trilipix, Antara, Fenoglide, Lipofen, Lofibra, Trilipix	Antihyperlipidemic, Fibric Acid Derivative
130	Gemfibrozil	Lopid	Antihyperlipidemic, Fibric Acid Derivative
131	Atorvastatin	Lipitor	Antihyperlipidemic, HMG-CoA Reductase Inhibitor
132	Lovastatin	Mevacor, Altoprev	Antihyperlipidemic, HMG-CoA Reductase Inhibitor
133	Pravastatin	Pravachol	Antihyperlipidemic, HMG-CoA Reductase Inhibitor
134	Rosuvastatin	Crestor	Antihyperlipidemic, HMG-CoA Reductase Inhibitor
135	Simvastatin	Zocor	Antihyperlipidemic, HMG-CoA Reductase Inhibitor
136	Lithium	Lithobid, Eskalith	Antimanic
137	Rizatriptan	Maxalt	Antimigraine, Serotonin Receptor Agonist
138	Sumatriptan	Imitrex	Antimigraine, Serotonin Receptor Agonist
139	Tamoxifen	Soltamox	Antineoplastic
140	Anastrozole	Arimidex	Antineoplastic, Aromatase Inhibitor
141	Carbidopa + Levodopa	Sinemet, Sinemet CR	Antiparkinson Agent
142	Benztropine	Cogentin	Antiparkinson Agent, Anticholinergic

#	GENERIC	BRAND	CLASS
143	Pramipexole	Mirapex	Antiparkinson Agent, Dopamine Agonist
144	Ropinirole	Requip	Antiparkinson Agent, Dopamine Agonist
145	Clopidogrel	Plavix	Antiplatelet
146	Aspirin	Ecotrin	Antiplatelet, NSAID, Salicylate
147	Haloperidol	Haldol	Antipsychotic
148	Lurasidone	Latuda	Antipsychotic
149	Ziprasidone	Geodon	Antipsychotic
150	Aripiprazole	Abilify	Antipsychotic, Antimanic
151	Olanzapine	Zyprexa	Antipsychotic, Antimanic
152	Quetiapine	Seroquel	Antipsychotic, Antimanic
153	Risperidone	Risperdal	Antipsychotic, Antimanic
154	Oxybutynin	Ditropan	Antispasmodic Agent, Urinary
155	Benzonatate	Tessalon Perles	Antitussive
156	Guaifenesin + Pseudoephedrine + Codeine	Cheratussin DAC, Virtussin DAC	Antitussive, Narcotic
157	Acyclovir	Zovirax	Antiviral
158	Oseltamivir	Tamiflu	Antiviral
159	Valacyclovir	Valtrex	Antiviral
160	Clonazepam	Klonopin	Benzodiazepines
161	Alprazolam	Xanax	Benzodiazepines, Antianxiety, Anxiolytic
162	Buspirone	Buspar	Benzodiazepines, Antianxiety, Anxiolytic
163	Lorazepam	Ativan	Benzodiazepines, Antianxiety, Anxiolytic, Sedative, Anticonvulsant
164	Diazepam	Valium	Benzodiazepines, Sedative
165	Mirabegron	Myrbetriq	Beta 3 Agonist
166	Atenolol	Tenormin	Beta Blocker
167	Bisoprolol	Zebeta	Beta Blocker
168	Carvedilol	Coreg	Beta Blocker
169	Labetalol	Normodyne	Beta Blocker
170	Metoprolol	Toprol XL, Lopressor	Beta Blocker

#	GENERIC	BRAND	CLASS
171	Nebivolol	Bystolic	Beta Blocker
172	Propranolol	Inderal	Beta Blocker
173	Atenolol + Chlorthalidone	Tenoretic	Beta Blocker + Diuretic
174	Metformin	Glucophage	Biguanide
175	Alendronate	Fosamax	Bisphosphonate
176	Albuterol	Proair HFA, Proventil HFA, Ventolin HFA	Bronchodilator
177	Ipratropium Bromide	Atrovent HFA	Bronchodilator
178	Tiotropium	Spiriva Handihaler	Bronchodilator
179	Amlodipine	Norvasc	Calcium Channel Blocker
180	Diltiazem	Cardizem, Cartia XT	Calcium Channel Blocker
181	Nifedipine	Procardia, Adalat	Calcium Channel Blocker
182	Verapamil	Calan SR	Calcium Channel Blocker
183	Amlodipine + Benazepril	Lotrel	Calcium Channel Blocker + Angiotensin-converting enzyme (ACE) Inhibitor
184	Donepezil	Aricept	Central Cholinesterase Inhibitor
185	Atomoxetine	Strattera	CNS Stimulant
186	Dexmethylphenidate Hydrochloride	Focalin	CNS Stimulant
187	Dextroamphetamine + Amphetamine	Adderall	CNS Stimulant
188	Lisdexamfetamine	Vyvanse	CNS stimulant
189	Methylphenidate	Ritalin, Concerta	CNS Stimulant
190	Phentermine	Adipex-P, Lomaira	CNS stimulant, appetite suppressant
191	Desogestrel + Ethinyl Estradiol	Apri, Cyclessa, Enskyce, Viorele	Contraceptive
192	Drospirenone + Ethinyl estradiol	Yaz	Contraceptive
193	Ethinyl Estradiol + Etonogestrel	NuvaRing	Contraceptive
194	Ethinyl Estradiol + Levonorgestrel	Twirla	Contraceptive
195	Ethinyl Estradiol + Norethindrone	Necon 777	Contraceptive
196	Ethinyl Estradiol + Norgestimate	Trinessa-28, Ortho Tri-Cyclen, Ortho Tri-Cyclen Lo	Contraceptive

#	GENERIC	BRAND	CLASS
197	Ethinyl Estradiol + Norgestrel	Cryselle	Contraceptive
198	Norethindrone	Errin, Heather, Camila	Contraceptive
199	Beclomethasone Dipropionate	Qvar	Corticosteroid
200	Budesonide	Pulmicort Flexhaler	Corticosteroid
201	Clobetasol	Impoyz, Temovate	Corticosteroid
202	Hydrocortisone Topical	Cortisone	Corticosteroid
203	Mometasone Nasal	Nasonex	Corticosteroid
204	Prednisone	Deltasone	Corticosteroid
205	Triamcinolone Topical	Kenalog, Trianex, Triacet, Nasacort AQ	Corticosteroid
206	Fluticasone + Salmeterol	Advair Diskus, Advair HFA	Corticosteroid + Beta Blocker
207	Betamethasone Dipropionate + Clotrimazole	Lotrisone	Corticosteroid, Antifungal
208	Methylprednisolone	Medrol	Corticosteroid, Anti-inflammatory
209	Sodium Chloride	Ocean, Ayr Saline	Decongestant, Intranasal
210	Linagliptin	Tradjenta	Dipeptidyl Peptidase IV Inhibitor
211	Bumetanide	Bumex, Burinex	Diuretic (Loop)
212	Furosemide	Lasix	Diuretic (Loop)
213	Torsemide	Demadex	Diuretic (Loop)
214	HCTZ + Triamterene	Dyazide, Maxzide	Diuretic (Potassium-sparing and Thiazide)
215	Spironolactone	Aldactone	Diuretic (Potassium-sparing)
216	Chlorthalidone	Hygroton, Thalitone	Diuretic (Thiazide)
217	Hydrochlorothiazide (HCTZ)	Microzide	Diuretic (Thiazide)
218	HCTZ + Losartan	Hyzaar	Diuretic + Angiotensin II Receptor Blocker
219	HCTZ + Olmesartan	Benicar HCT	Diuretic + Angiotensin II Receptor Blocker
220	HCTZ + Valsartan	Diovan HCT	Diuretic + Angiotensin II Receptor Blocker
221	Hydrochlorothiazide (HCTZ) + Lisinopril	Zestoretic	Diuretic + Angiotensin-converting enzyme (ACE) Inhibitor
222	Adalimumab	Humira	DMARD, Antipsoriatic
223	Potassium Chloride	Klor-Con	Electrolyte Supplements

#	GENERIC	BRAND	CLASS
224	Estradiol oral	Estrace	Estrogen Derivatives
225	Estrogens, Conjugated	Premarin	Estrogen Derivatives
226	Guaifenesin	Mucinex	Expectorant
227	Sucralfate	Carafate	Gastrointestinal Agent
228	Linaclotide	Linzess	Gastrointestinal, IBS Agent
229	Dulaglutide	Trulicity	Glucagon-Like Peptide-1 Receptor Agonist
230	Exenatide	Byetta, Bydureon	Glucagon-Like Peptide-1 Receptor Agonist
231	Liraglutide	Victoza, Saxenda	Glucagon-Like Peptide-1 Receptor Agonist
232	Prednisolone Oral	Orapred, Prelone, Pediapred	Glucocorticosteroid
233	Famotidine	Pepcid	Histamine H2 Antagoist
234	Ranitidine	Zantac	Histamine H2 Antagoist
235	Emtricitabine	Emtriva	HIV, NRTI
236	Conjugated Estrogens + Medroxyprogesterone	Prempro	Hormone Replacement
237	Mycophenolate	CellCept, Myfortic	Immunosuppressant
238	Methotrexate	Trexall	Immunosuppressant, Antineoplstic, DMARD
239	Cyclosporine	Neoral, Sandimmune, Gengraf	Immunosuppressant, DMARD, Calcineurin Inhibitor
240	Fluticasone	Flonase, Veramyst, Flovent HFA, Arnuity Ellipta, Flovent Diskus	Intranasal Adrenal Glucocorticosteroid
241	Ferrous Sulfate	Feosol, Fer-In-Sol	Iron Product
242	Docusate Sodium	Colace	Laxative
243	Methylcellulose	Citrucel	Laxative
244	Polyethylene Glycol 3350	Golytely	Laxative
245	Sennosides	Senna, Senokot	Laxative
246	Montelukast	Singulair	Leukotriene Inhibitor
247	Lidocaine Patch	Lidoderm	Local Anesthetic
248	Isosorbide Mononitrate	Imdur	Nitrate
249	Nitroglycerin	Nitrostat, Minitran	Nitrate, Vasodilator
250	Memantine	Namenda	NMDA Antagonist
251	Celecoxib	Celebrex	Nonsteroidal anti-inflammatory drugs (NSAID)

#	GENERIC	BRAND	CLASS
252	Diclofenac Sodium	Voltaren, Cambia, Zipsor, Zorvolex	Nonsteroidal anti-inflammatory drugs (NSAID)
253	Ibuprofen	Motrin, Advil	Nonsteroidal anti-inflammatory drugs (NSAID)
254	Indomethacin	Indocin, Tivorbex	Nonsteroidal anti-inflammatory drugs (NSAID)
255	Ketorolac	Toradol	Nonsteroidal anti-inflammatory drugs (NSAID)
256	Meloxicam	Mobic	Nonsteroidal anti-inflammatory drugs (NSAID)
257	Naproxen	Anaprox	Nonsteroidal anti-inflammatory drugs (NSAID)
258	Buprenorphine + Naloxone	Suboxone, Bunavail, Zubsolv	Opioid partial agonist and antagonist combination
259	Sodium Fluoride	PreviDent	Oral Rinse
260	Pancrelipase	Creon, Zenpep	Pancreatic/Digestive Enzyme
261	Hydralazine	Apresoline	Peripheral Vasodilator
262	Sildenafil	Viagra, Revatio	Phosphodiesterase-5 (PDE-5) Enzyme Inhibitor
263	Tadalafil	Cialis	Phosphodiesterase-5 (PDE-5) Enzyme Inhibitor
264	Medroxyprogesterone	Provera, Depo-Provera	Progestin hormone
265	Progesterone	Prometrium	Progestin Hormone
266	Latanoprost	Xalatan	Prostaglandin
267	Dexlansoprazole	Dexilant	Proton Pump Inhibitor
268	Esomeprazole	Nexium	Proton Pump Inhibitor
269	Lansoprazole	Prevacid	Proton Pump Inhibitor
270	Omeprazole	Prilosec	Proton Pump Inhibitor
271	Rabeprazole	Aciphex	Proton Pump Inhibitor
272	Pantoprazole	Protonix	Proton Pump Inhibitor
273	Albuterol Sulfate + Ipratropium Bromide	Combivent Respimat	Respiratory Inhalant Combo
274	Budesonide + Formoterol	Symbicort	Respiratory Inhalant Combo
275	Formoterol + Mometasone	Dulera	Respiratory Inhalant Combos, Bronchodilator
276	Eszopiclone	Lunesta	Sedative
277	Temazepam	Restoril	Sedative, Hypnotic
278	Triazolam	Halcion	Sedative, Hypnotic

#	GENERIC	BRAND	CLASS
279	Zolpidem	Ambien, Ambien CR, Intermezzo	Sedative, Hypnotic
280	Desvenlafaxine	Pristiq, Khedezla	Serotonin/Norepinephrine Reuptake Inhibitor
281	Duloxetine	Cymbalta	Serotonin/Norepinephrine Reuptake Inhibitor
282	Baclofen	Lioresal	Skeletal Muscle Relaxant
283	Carisoprodol	Soma	Skeletal Muscle Relaxant
284	Cyclobenzaprine	Flexeril	Skeletal Muscle Relaxant
285	Methocarbamol	Robaxin	Skeletal Muscle Relaxant
286	Canagliflozin	Invokana	Sodium-glucose cotransporter 2 inhibitor
287	Dapagliflozin	Farxiga	Sodium-glucose cotransporter 2 inhibitor
288	Levothyroxine	Synthroid	Thyroid
289	Liothyronine	Cytomel, Triostat	Thyroid
290	Methimazole	Tapazole	Thyroid
291	Thyroid	Armour Thyroid	Thyroid
292	Colchicine	Colcrys	Uricosuric Agent
293	Calcitriol	Rocaltrol	Vitamin D Analogs
294	Calcium + Cholecalciferol	Os-Cal Ultra, Caltrate 600 + D3	Vitamin, Fat-Soluble
295	Ergocalciferol	Vitamin D	Vitamins, Fat-Soluble
296	Cyanocobalamin	Vitamin B12	Vitamins, Water-Soluble
297	Folic Acid	Folate, Folvite	Vitamins, Water-Soluble
298	Allopurinol	Zyloprim	Xanthine Oxidase Inhibitor
299	Clonidine	Catapres	α2-Adrenergic Agonist
300	Guanfacine	Intuniv	α2-Adrenergic Agonist

By Brand (Top 300)

#	BRAND	GENERIC
1	Abilify	Aripiprazole
2	Accupril	Quinapril
3	Aciphex	Rabeprazole
4	Actos	Pioglitazone
5	Adderall	Dextroamphetamine + Amphetamine
6	Adipex-P, Lomaira	Phentermine
7	Advair Diskus, Advair HFA	Fluticasone + Salmeterol
8	Aldactone	Spironolactone
9	Allegra	Fexofenadine
10	Alphagan P	Brimonidine tartrate
11	Altace	Ramipril
12	Amaryl	Glimepiride
13	Ambien, Ambien CR, Intermezzo	Zolpidem
14	Amoxil	Amoxicillin
15	Anaprox	Naproxen
16	Androgel, Androderm	Testosterone
17	Antivert, Bonine, Dramamine	Meclizine
18	Apresoline	Hydralazine
19	Apri, Cyclessa, Enskyce, Viorele	Desogestrel + Ethinyl Estradiol
20	Aricept	Donepezil
21	Arimidex	Anastrozole
22	Armour Thyroid	Thyroid
23	Asacol	Mesalamine
24	Astelin, Astepro	Azelastine
25	Atarax, Vistaril	Hydroxyzine
26	Ativan	Lorazepam
27	Atrovent HFA	Ipratropium Bromide
28	Augmentin	Amoxicillin + Clavulanate
29	Avapro	Irbesartan

#	BRAND	GENERIC
30	Avodart	Dutasteride
31	Bactrim	Sulfamethoxazole + Trimethoprim
32	Bactroban	Mupirocin
33	Benadryl	Diphenhydramine
34	Bengay Cold Therapy, Icy Hot Naturals	Menthol
35	Benicar	Olmesartan
36	Benicar HCT	HCTZ + Olmesartan
37	Bentyl	Dicyclomine
38	Betapace, Sorine	Sotalol
39	Bumex, Burinex	Bumetanide
40	Buspar	Buspirone
41	Byetta, Bydureon	Exenatide
42	Bystolic	Nebivolol
43	Calan SR	Verapamil
44	Carafate	Sucralfate
45	Cardizem, Cartia XT	Diltiazem
46	Cardura, Cardura-XL	Doxazosin
47	Catapres	Clonidine
48	Celebrex	Celecoxib
49	Celexa	Citalopram
50	CellCept, Myfortic	Mycophenolate
51	Cheratussin DAC, Virtussin DAC	Guaifenesin + Pseudoephedrine + Codeine
52	Cialis	Tadalafil
53	Cipro	Ciprofloxacin Oral
54	Citrucel	Methylcellulose
55	Claritin, Alavert	Loratadine
56	Cleocin	Clindamycin
57	Cogentin	Benztropine
58	Colace	Docusate Sodium
59	Colcrys	Colchicine
60	Combivent Respimat	Albuterol Sulfate + Ipratropium Bromide
61	Cordarone	Amiodarone

#	BRAND	GENERIC
62	Coreg	Carvedilol
63	Cortisone	Hydrocortisone Topical
64	Cosopt	Dorzolamide + Timolol
65	Coumadin	Warfarin
66	Cozaar	Losartan
67	Creon, Zenpep	Pancrelipase
68	Crestor	Rosuvastatin
69	Cryselle	Ethinyl Estradiol + Norgestrel
70	Cymbalta	Duloxetine
71	Cytomel, Triostat	Liothyronine
72	Deltasone	Prednisone
73	Demadex	Torsemide
74	Depakote, Depakote ER	Divalproex
75	Desyrel	Trazodone
76	Detrol LA	Tolterodine
77	Dexilant	Dexlansoprazole
78	Diflucan	Fluconazole
79	Dilantin	Phenytoin
80	Dilaudid	Hydromorphone
81	Diovan	Valsartan
82	Diovan HCT	HCTZ + Valsartan
83	Ditropan	Oxybutynin
84	Drenaclick, Auvi-Q, EpiPen, EpiPen Jr	Epinephrine Auto-Injector
85	Dulera	Formoterol + Mometasone
86	Duragesic Patch, Lonsys	Fentanyl
87	Dyazide, Maxzide	HCTZ + Triamterene
88	Dynacin, Minocin, Solodyn	Minocycline
89	Ecotrin	Aspirin
90	Effexor	Venlafaxine
91	Elavil	Amitriptyline
92	Eliquis	Apixaban
93	Emtriva	Emtricitabine

#	BRAND	GENERIC
94	Errin, Heather, Camila	Norethindrone
95	Erythrocin	Erythromycin
96	Estrace	Estradiol oral
97	Farxiga	Dapagliflozin
98	Feosol, Fer-In-Sol	Ferrous Sulfate
99	Flagyl	Metronidazole
100	Flexeril	Cyclobenzaprine
101	Flomax	Tamsulosin
102	Flonase, Veramyst, Flovent HFA, Arnuity Ellipta, Flovent Diskus	Fluticasone
103	Focalin	Dexmethylphenidate Hydrochloride
104	Folate, Folvite	Folic Acid
105	Fosamax	Alendronate
106	Geodon	Ziprasidone
107	Glucophage	Metformin
108	Glucotrol	Glipizide
109	Golytely	Polyethylene Glycol 3350
110	Halcion	Triazolam
111	Haldol	Haloperidol
112	Humalog	Insulin Lispro
113	Humira	Adalimumab
114	Humulin R, Novolin R	Insulin Human
115	Hygroton, Thalitone	Chlorthalidone
116	Hytrin	Terazosin
117	Hyzaar	HCTZ + Losartan
118	Imdur	Isosorbide Mononitrate
119	Imitrex	Sumatriptan
120	Impoyz, Temovate	Clobetasol
121	Inderal	Propranolol
122	Indocin, Tivorbex	Indomethacin
123	Intuniv	Guanfacine
124	Invokana	Canagliflozin

#	BRAND	GENERIC
125	Janumet XR	Metformin + Sitagliptin
126	Januvia	Sitagliptin
127	Jardiance	Empagliflozin
128	Keflex	Cephalexin
129	Kenalog, Trianex, Triacet, Nasacort AQ	Triamcinolone Topical
130	Keppra	Levetiracetam
131	Klonopin	Clonazepam
132	Klor-Con	Potassium Chloride
133	Lamictal	Lamotrigine
134	Lanoxin	Digoxin
135	Lantus	Insulin Glargine
136	Lasix	Furosemide
137	Latuda	Lurasidone
138	Levaquin	Levofloxacin
139	Levemir	Insulin Detemir
140	Lexapro	Escitalopram
141	Lidoderm	Lidocaine Patch
142	Linzess	Linaclotide
143	Lioresal	Baclofen
144	Lipitor	Atorvastatin
145	Lithobid, Eskalith	Lithium
146	Lopid	Gemfibrozil
147	Lotensin	Benazepril
148	Lotrel	Amlodipine + Benazepril
149	Lotrisone	Betamethasone Dipropionate + Clotrimazole
150	Lovaza	Omega-3 Fatty Acid Ethyl Esters
151	Lovenox	Enoxaparin
152	Lumigan	Bimatoprost
153	Lunesta	Eszopiclone
154	Lyrica	Pregabalin
155	Macrobid, Macrodantin	Nitrofurantoin
156	Mag-Ox 400	Magnesium Oxide

#	BRAND	GENERIC
157	Maxalt	Rizatriptan
158	Medrol	Methylprednisolone
159	Mevacor, Altoprev	Lovastatin
160	Micardis	Telmisartan
161	Micronase, Diabeta	Glyburide
162	Microzide	Hydrochlorothiazide (HCTZ)
163	Minipress, Prazo, Prazin	Prazosin
164	Mirapex	Pramipexole
165	Mobic	Meloxicam
166	Motrin, Advil	Ibuprofen
167	MS Contin, Avinza, Kadian	Morphine Sulfate
168	Mucinex	Guaifenesin
169	Mycostatin, Nyamyc, Nystop	Nystatin
170	Myrbetriq	Mirabegron
171	Mysoline	Primidone
172	Namenda	Memantine
173	Naphcon-A, Opcon-A, Visine-A	Naphazoline + Pheniramine
174	Nasonex	Mometasone Nasal
175	Necon 777	Ethinyl Estradiol + Norethindrone
176	Neoral, Sandimmune, Gengraf	Cyclosporine
177	Neosporin	Bacitracin + Neomycin + Polymyxin B
178	Neurontin	Gabapentin
179	Nexium	Esomeprazole
180	Niaspan, Slo-Niacin	Niacin
181	Nitrostat, Minitran	Nitroglycerin
182	Nizoral	Ketoconazole Topical
183	Norco, Vicodin, Lorcet	Acetaminophen + Hydrocodone
184	Normodyne	Labetalol
185	Norvasc	Amlodipine
186	Novolog	Insulin Aspart
187	NuvaRing	Ethinyl Estradiol + Etonogestrel
188	Ocean, Ayr Saline	Sodium Chloride

#	BRAND	GENERIC
189	Ocuflox	Ofloxacin
190	Omnicef	Cefdinir
191	Orapred, Prelone, Pediapred	Prednisolone Oral
192	Os-Cal Ultra, Caltrate 600 + D3	Calcium + Cholecalciferol
193	OxyContin	Oxycodone
194	Pamelor	Nortriptyline
195	Patanol, Pataday	Olopatadine
196	Paxil	Paroxetine
197	Pen Vee K, Penicillin V	Penicillin VK
198	Pepcid	Famotidine
199	Peridex, PerioGard, PerioChip	Chlorhexidine
200	Phenergan	Promethazine
201	Phrenilin Forte, Phrenilin, Bupap, Orbivan CF	Acetaminophen + Butalbital
202	Plaquenil	Hydroxychloroquine
203	Plavix	Clopidogrel
204	Pravachol	Pravastatin
205	Premarin	Estrogens, Conjugated
206	Prempro	Conjugated Estrogens + Medroxyprogesterone
207	Prevacid	Lansoprazole
208	PreviDent	Sodium Fluoride
209	Prilosec	Omeprazole
210	Prinivil, Zestril	Lisinopril
211	Pristiq, Khedezla	Desvenlafaxine
212	Proair HFA, Proventil HFA, Ventolin HFA	Albuterol
213	Procardia, Adalat	Nifedipine
214	Prometrium	Progesterone
215	Proscar, Propecia	Finasteride
216	Protonix	Pantoprazole
217	Provera, Depo-Provera	Medroxyprogesterone
218	Prozac	Fluoxetine
219	Pulmicort Flexhaler	Budesonide

#	BRAND	GENERIC
220	Qvar	Beclomethasone Dipropionate
221	Ranexa	Ranolazine
222	Reglan	Metoclopramide
223	Remeron	Mirtazapine
224	Requip	Ropinirole
225	Restoril	Temazepam
226	Retin A	Tretinoin
227	Risperdal	Risperidone
228	Ritalin, Concerta	Methylphenidate
229	Robaxin	Methocarbamol
230	Rocaltrol	Calcitriol
231	Senna, Senokot	Sennosides
232	Seroquel	Quetiapine
233	Sinemet, Sinemet CR	Carbidopa + Levodopa
234	Sinequan, Silenor	Doxepin
235	Singulair	Montelukast
236	Soltamox	Tamoxifen
237	Soma	Carisoprodol
238	Spiriva Handihaler	Tiotropium
239	Strattera	Atomoxetine
240	Suboxone, Bunavail, Zubsolv	Buprenorphine + Naloxone
241	Symbicort	Budesonide + Formoterol
242	Synthroid	Levothyroxine
243	Tambacor	Flecainide
244	Tamiflu	Oseltamivir
245	Tapazole	Methimazole
246	Tegretol	Carbamazepine
247	Tenoretic	Atenolol + Chlorthalidone
248	Tenormin	Atenolol
249	Tessalon Perles	Benzonatate
250	Timoptic	Timolol
251	Topamax	Topiramate

#	BRAND	GENERIC
252	Toprol XL, Lopressor	Metoprolol
253	Toradol	Ketorolac
254	Tradjenta	Linagliptin
255	Travatan Z	Travoprost
256	Tresiba	Insulin Degludec
257	Trexall	Methotrexate
258	Tricor, Trilipix, Antara, Fenoglide, Lipofen, Lofibra, Trilipix	Fenofibrate
259	Trileptal	Oxcarbazepine
260	Trinessa-28, Ortho Tri-Cyclen, Ortho Tri-Cyclen Lo	Ethinyl Estradiol + Norgestimate
261	Trulicity	Dulaglutide
262	Trusopt	Dorzolamide
263	Tums, Oysco	Calcium
264	Twirla	Ethinyl Estradiol + Levonorgestrel
265	Tylenol	Acetaminophen
266	Ultram	Tramadol
267	Uroxatral	Alfuzosin
268	Valium	Diazepam
269	Valtrex	Valacyclovir
270	Vasotec	Enalapril
271	Vesicare	Solifenacin
272	Viagra, Revatio	Sildenafil
273	Vibramycin	Doxycycline
274	Victoza, Saxenda	Liraglutide
275	Viibryd	Vilazodone
276	Vitamin B12	Cyanocobalamin
277	Vitamin D	Ergocalciferol
278	Voltaren, Cambia, Zipsor, Zorvolex	Diclofenac Sodium
279	Vytorin	Ezetimibe + Simvastatin
280	Vyvanse	Lisdexamfetamine
281	Wellbutrin, Zyban	Bupropion
282	Xalatan	Latanoprost

#	BRAND	GENERIC
283	Xanax	Alprazolam
284	Xarelto	Rivaroxaban
285	Xyzal	Levocetirizine
286	Yaz	Drospirenone + Ethinyl estradiol
287	Zanaflex	Tizanidine
288	Zantac	Ranitidine
289	Zebeta	Bisoprolol
290	Zestoretic	Hydrochlorothiazide (HCTZ) + Lisinopril
291	Zetia	Ezetimibe
292	Zocor	Simvastatin
293	Zofran	Ondansetron
294	Zohydro ER, Hysingla ER, Vantrela ER	Hydrocodone Bitartrate
295	Zoloft	Sertraline
296	Zovirax	Acyclovir
297	Z-Pak, Zithromax	Azithromycin
298	Zyloprim	Allopurinol
299	Zyprexa	Olanzapine
300	Zyrtec	Cetirizine

Extra Practice 100 Medications

#	GENERIC	BRAND
1	Adapalene	Differin
2	Abacavir + Lamivudine	Epzicom
3	Acetaminophen + Codeine	Tylenol with Codeine
4	Acetaminophen + Oxycodone	Percocet
5	Acetaminophen + Tramadol	Ultracet
6	Aliskiren	Tekturna
7	Amlodipine + Olmesartan	Azor
8	Amlodipine + Valsartan	Exforge
9	Atazanavir	Reyataz
10	Azathioprine	Azamun, Imuran
11	Benzoyl Peroxide + Clindamycin	Benzaclin
12	Butalbital + Caffeine + Acetaminophen	Fioricet
13	Butalbital + Caffeine + Aspirin	Fiorinal
14	Candesartan	Atacand
15	Candesartan + HCTZ	Atacand-HCT
16	Captopril	Capoten
17	Cefaclor	Ceclor
18	Cefazolin	Ancef
19	Cefprozil	Cefzil
20	Cefuroxime	Ceftin
21	Cinacalcet	Sensipar
22	Ciprofloxacin + Dexamethasone Otic (Ear Drop)	Ciprodex
23	Clarithromycin	Biaxin
24	Clobazam	Onfi
25	Clorazepate	Tranxene-T
26	Colesevelam	Welchol
27	Dabigatran	Pradaxa
28	Dexamethasone	Decadron
29	Diphenoxylate and Atropine	Lomotil

#	GENERIC	BRAND
30	Efavirenz	Sustiva
31	Eletriptan	Relpax
32	Elmisartan + HCTZ	Micardis-HCT
33	Emtricitabine + Tenofovir	Truvada
34	Entecavir	Baraclude
35	Etodolac	Lodine
36	Febuxostat	Uloric
37	Felodipine	Plendil
38	Fexofenadine + Pseudoephedrine	Allegra-D
39	Fluocinonide Topical	Lidex
40	Fluvoxamine	Luvox
41	Fosinopril	Monopril
42	Gatifloxacin	Zymar, Zymaxid
43	Hepatitis A Vaccine	Havrix, Vaqta
44	Hepatitis B Vaccine	Engerix-B, Recombivax HB
45	Herpes Zoster Vaccine	Zostavax, Shingrix
46	Human Papillomavirus Vaccine	Gardasil 9
47	Hydrocodone + Ibuprofen	Vicoprofen
48	Ibandronate	Boniva
49	Imiquimod	Zyclara, Aldara
50	Influenza Vaccine	Afluria, Fluad, Fluzone, Fluarix
51	Insulin Aspart Protamine (70%), Aspart (30%)	NovoLog Mix 70/30
52	Insulin Glulisine	Apidra
53	Insulin NPH	Humulin N, Novolin N
54	Insulin NPH (70%),	Humulin 70/30,
55	Irbesartan + HCTZ	Avalide
56	Isotretinoin	Zenatane
57	Lacosamide	Vimpat
58	Levalbuterol	Xopenex HFA
59	Loteprednol	Alrex, Lotemax
60	Lubiprostone	Amitiza

#	GENERIC	BRAND
61	Maraviroc	Selzentry
62	Measles, Mumps, Rubella Vaccine	MMR-II
63	Meningococcal Vaccine	Menactra, Menveo Trumenba, Bexero
64	Meperidine	Demerol
65	Methadone	Dolophine
66	Methylprednisolone	Medrol
67	Moxifloxacin	Vigamox,
68	Nabumetone	Relafen
69	Nateglinide	Starlix
70	Perindopril	Aceon
71	Phenazopyridine	Pyridium
72	Phenobarbital	Luminal
73	Piroxicam	Feldene
74	Pneumococcal Vaccine	Prevnar 13, Pneumovax 23
75	Polio Vaccine	Ipol
76	Prochlorperazine	Compazine
77	Raloxifene	Evista
78	Raltegravir	Isentress
79	Ramelteon	Rozerem
80	Regular (30%)	Novolin 70/30
81	Repaglinide	Prandin
82	Rifaximin	Xifaxan
83	Risedronate	Actonel, Atelvia
84	Rosiglitazone	Avandia
85	Rotavirus Vaccine	Rotarix, RotaTeq
86	Sacubitril + Valsartan	Entresto
87	Saxagliptin	Onglyza
88	Scopolamine	Transdermscop
89	Sevelamer carbonate	Renvela
90	Tacrolimus	Prograf
91	Tdap (Tetanus, Diphtheria, Pertussis)	Daptacel, Adacel, Boostrix, Infanrix
92	Terbinafine	Lamisil

#	GENERIC	BRAND
93	Ticagrelor	Brilinta
94	Tobramycin	Tobrex
95	Tropium	Sanctura
96	Vancomycin	Vancocin
97	Vardenafil	Levitra
98	Varenicline	Chantix
99	Zaleplon	Sonata
100	Zolmitriptan	Zomig

INDEX

D

Dabigatran 107
Dapagliflozin 25, 56, 83, 119, 131
Daptacel 106
Decadron 104
Degludec 24, 62, 91, 119, 124
Deltasone 47, 68, 82, 134
Demadex 20, 70, 82, 134
Demerol 105
Depakote 35, 57, 82, 134
Depo-Provera 30, 64, 90, 138
Desogestrel 29, 56, 79, 116, 128
Desvenlafaxine 44, 56, 89, 118, 130
Desyrel 44, 71, 82, 134
Detemir 24, 62, 85, 114, 125
Detrol 50, 70, 82, 134
Dexamethasone 103, 104
Dexilant 28, 57, 82, 134
Dexlansoprazole 28, 57, 82, 117, 130
Dexmethylphenidate 44, 57, 83, 117, 127
Dextroamphetamine 44, 57, 78, 112, 127
Diabeta 25, 61, 87, 137
Diazepam 36, 57, 92, 115, 127
Diclofenac 36, 57, 93, 114, 129
Dicyclomine 28, 57, 80, 117, 123
Differin 102
Diflucan 32, 60, 82, 134
Digoxin 19, 57, 85, 116, 123
Dilantin 35, 67, 82, 134
Dilaudid 37, 61, 82, 134
Diltiazem 18, 57, 80, 113, 127
Diovan 18, 61, 71, 82, 134
Diphenhydramine 48, 57, 80, 119, 125
Diphenoxylate 107
Ditropan 50, 67, 82, 134
Divalproex 35, 57, 82, 115, 124
Docusate 27, 57, 81, 115, 129
Dolophine 105
Donepezil 35, 57, 79, 115, 127
Dorzolamide 41, 57, 81, 92, 118, 120,
125
Doxazosin 49, 58, 80, 116, 122
Doxepin 44, 58, 90, 119, 124
Doxycycline 22, 58, 92, 114, 123
Dramamine 27, 64, 79, 132
Drenaclick 21, 58, 82, 134
Drospirenone 29, 58, 93, 114, 128
Dulaglutide 25, 58, 92, 118, 129
Dulera 47, 60, 82, 134
Duloxetine 44, 58, 82, 112, 130
DuoNeb 47
Duragesic 37, 60, 82, 134
Dutasteride 50, 58, 80, 120, 122
Dyazide 20, 61, 83, 134
Dynacin 22, 65, 83, 134

E

Ecotrin 36, 53, 83, 134
Efavirenz 103
Effexor 44, 71, 83, 134
Elavil 44, 53, 83, 134
Eletriptan 104
Eliquis 19, 53, 83, 134
Elmisartan 103
Empagliflozin 24, 58, 85, 118, 125
Emtricitabine 33, 58, 83, 103, 118, 129
Emtriva 33, 58, 83, 135
Enalapril 17, 58, 92, 115, 123
Engerix-B 106
Enoxaparin 19, 58, 86, 121, 124
Enskyce 29, 56, 79, 132
Entecavir 103
Entresto 104
Epinephrine 21, 58, 82, 119, 122
EpiPen 21, 58, 82, 134
Epzicom 103
Ergocalciferol 38, 58, 93, 112, 131
Errin 29, 66, 83, 135
Erythrocin 22, 58, 83, 135

M

U

W

V

X

Y

Z

ACKNOWLEDGEMENTS

I wanted to start with a special thanks to Linda Chang for her continual support and belief in me. Without her constant reminder for me to keep going and never stop taking small steps, this book wouldn't have existed. She knows how much I want to help those who need guidance on passing their exams and advancing in their careers.

Many thanks to William Peralta, Priscilla Valenzuela, Gustavo Hernandez, Daisy Ramirez, Kristin Camargo, Jasmine Mena, Diana Marquez, Jessica Marin, Janet Juarez, Monica Velasquez, Christina Montalvo, Martha Reynoso, and many other pharmacy technicians I have worked with at CVS pharmacy for their input on ways to become a licensed pharmacy technician and the types of resources they wish they had as they prepared for their PTCB exam. They justified my decision to put these medications together in a simplified manner, making them easy to quickly memorize.

I am grateful for the support and words of encouragement from Cindy Lin and my previous co-author, Kathy Chow. Thanks for cheering me up when I really needed it and for rekindling my belief in personal power to achieve one's dreams.

Last but not least, I wouldn't be able to write this book without the unconditional love from my parents. I can never thank them enough. To the many friends, colleagues, and brothers from Kappa Psi Pharmaceutical Fraternity whose input also helped to shape the content of this book.

ABOUT THE AUTHOR

Ryan Ngov, PharmD graduated from Western University of Health Sciences and founded Reshape The Mind, Inc., a consulting company that provides mentoring services, academic counseling, and career guidance for high school and college students. He is an expert at taking even high achievers to greater levels of success, which is evidenced by their acceptance into Stanford, Brown, UCLA, and other highly competitive colleges, graduate schools, and professional schools across the United States.

REFERENCES

ASHP Online Directory. https://accreditation.ashp.org/directory/#/program/ technician. Accessed 21 Sept. 2020.

Board of Pharmacy, California. "Pharmacy Technician License - California State Board of Pharmacy." *CA.Gov*, https://www.pharmacy.ca.gov/ applicants/tch.shtml. Accessed 10 July. 2020.

"Choose PTCB. Choose Excellence." *PTCB*, https://www.ptcb.org/guidebook/ ptce-content-outline#ptce-content-outline. Accessed 18 Sept. 2020.

"Choose PTCB. Choose Excellence." *PTCB*, https://www.ptcb.org/credentials/ certified-pharmacy-technician. Accessed 19 Sept. 2020.

"Drug, OTCs & Herbals | Medscape Reference." *Http://Reference.Medscape.Com*, http://reference.medscape.com/drugs. Accessed 9 Jul. 2020.

Drug Information Portal - U.S. National Library of Medicine - Quick Access to Quality Drug Information. https://druginfo.nlm.nih.gov/drugportal/. Accessed 4 Aug. 2020.

Horsley, K. (2016). *Unlimited memory: How to use advanced learning strategies to learn faster, remember more and be more productive.* TCK Publishing.

Kane, Sean. "The Top 300 of 2020." *Clincalc.Com*, 11 Feb. 2017, https://clincalc. com/DrugStats/Top300Drugs.aspx. Accessed 6 Sept. 2020.

"Lexicomp Online for Community Pharmacy." *Clinical Drug Information*, 9 July 2020, https://www.wolterskluwercdi.com/lexicomp-online/ community-pharmacy/. Accessed 2 Jun. 2020.

Mizner, J. J. (2020). *Mosby's pharmacy technician exam review.* St. Louis, MO: Elsevier/ Mosby.

NHA Certification Frequently Asked Questions. http://www.nhanow.com/help-center/faq. Accessed 19 Sept. 2020.

Salley, Jessica. *The ExCPT Exam — What to Expect and How to Prepare.* https://info.nhanow.com/blog/the-excpt-exam-what-to-expect-and-how-to-prepare. Accessed 18 Sept. 2020.

"Technician Program Accreditation - ASHP." *ASHP ASHP,* https://www.ashp.org/Professional-Development/Technician-Program-Accreditation. Accessed 19 Sept. 2020.

"The Top 200 Drugs of 2017?" *Pharmacy Times,* https://www.pharmacytimes.com/contributor/tony-guerra-pharmd/2017/03/the-top-200-drugs-of-2017. Accessed 3 Aug. 2020.

"View Document - California Code of Regulations." *Thomson Reuters Westlaw,* https://bit.ly/3cccLlP. Accessed 1 Sept. 2020.

Wells, B. G., Schwinghammer, T. L., DiPiro, J. T., & DiPiro, C. V. (2017). *Pharmacotherapy handbook.* New York: McGraw-Hill Education.